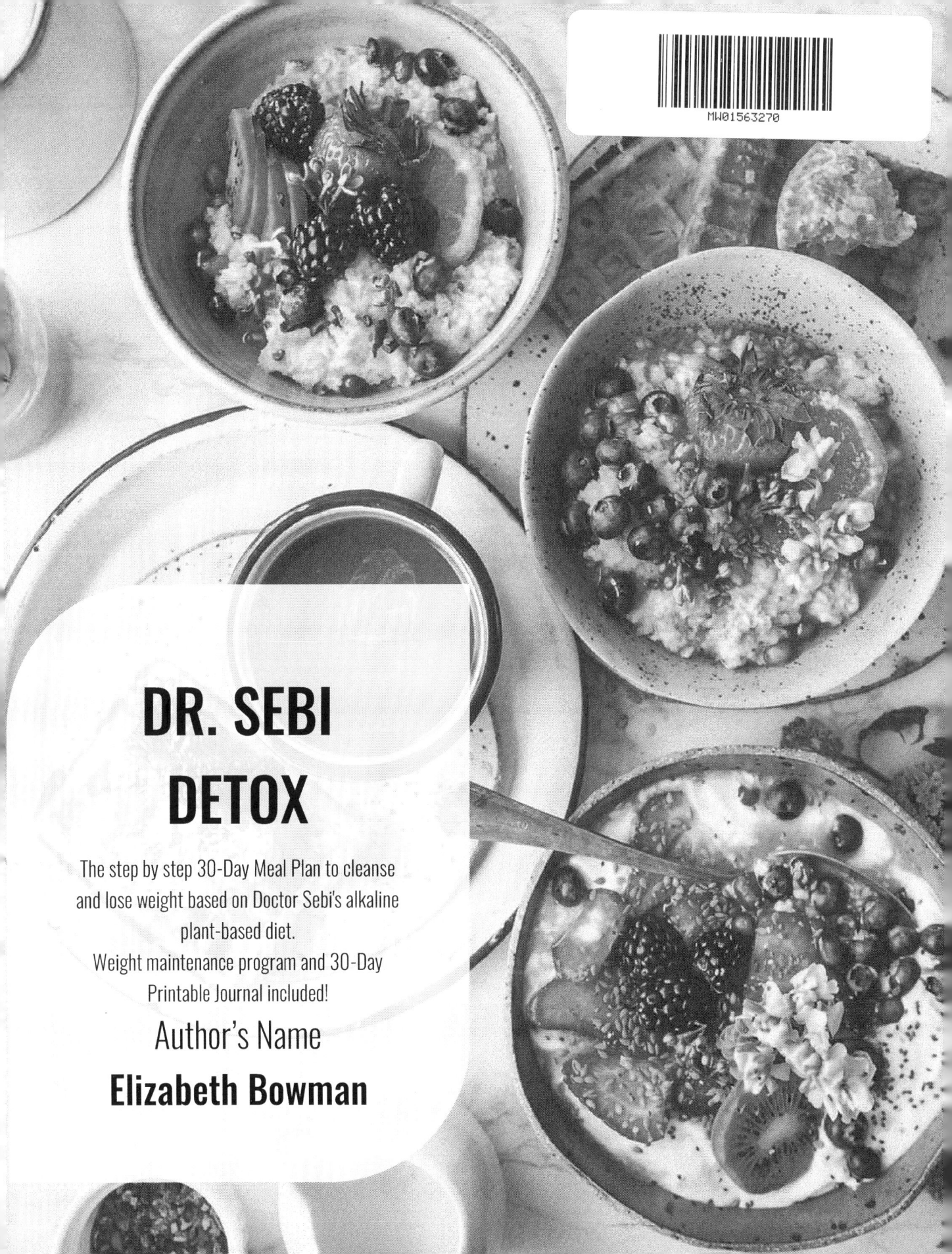

DR. SEBI DETOX

The step by step 30-Day Meal Plan to cleanse and lose weight based on Doctor Sebi's alkaline plant-based diet.
Weight maintenance program and 30-Day Printable Journal included!

Author's Name
Elizabeth Bowman

© Copyright 2021 by *Elizabeth Bowman* All rights reserved.

This document is geared towards providing exact and reliable information with regards to the topic and issue covered. The publication is sold with the idea that the publisher is not required to render accounting, officially permitted, or otherwise, qualified services. If advice is necessary, legal or professional, a practiced individual in the profession should be ordered.

- From a Declaration of Principles which was accepted and approved equally by a Committee of the American Bar Association and a Committee of Publishers and Associations.

In no way is it legal to reproduce, duplicate, or transmit any part of this document in either electronic means or in printed format. Recording of this publication is strictly prohibited and any storage of this document is not allowed unless with written permission from the publisher. All rights reserved.

The information provided herein is stated to be truthful and consistent, in that any liability, in terms of inattention or otherwise, by any usage or abuse of any policies, processes, or directions contained within is the solitary and utter responsibility of the recipient reader. Under no circumstances will any legal responsibility or blame be held against the publisher for any reparation, damages, or monetary loss due to the information herein, either directly or indirectly.

Respective authors own all copyrights not held by the publisher.

The information herein is offered for informational purposes solely, and is universal as so. The presentation of the information is without contract or any type of guarantee assurance.

The trademarks that are used are without any consent, and the publication of the trademark is without permission or backing by the trademark owner. All trademarks and brands within this book are for clarifying purposes only and are the owned by the owners themselves, not affiliated with this document

THIS BOOK INCLUDES

The diary

Dr. Sebi Journal

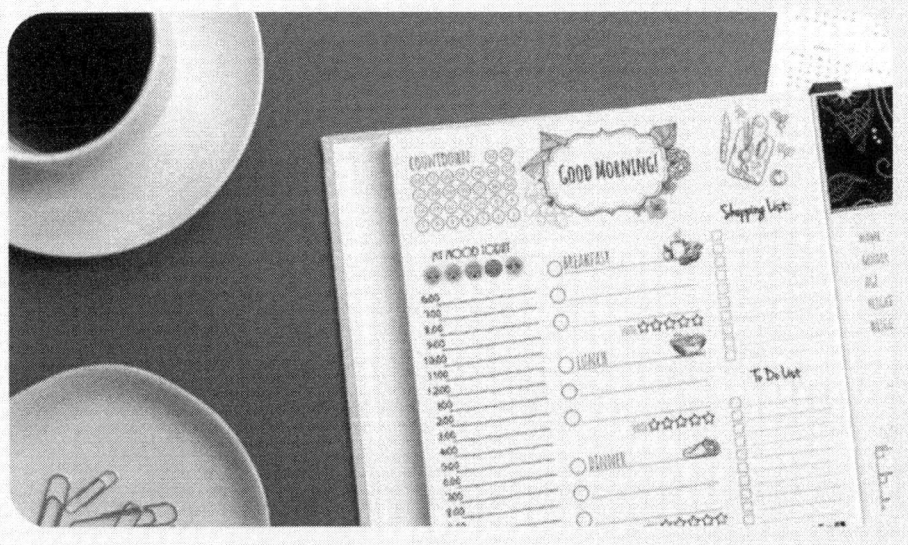

FILLABLE AND PRINTABLE ONLINE VERSION!!!

THE FOOD AND MOTIVATIONAL DIARY, **MADE EXCLUSIVELY FOR THIS BOOK**

TABLE OF CONTENTS

INTRODUCTION 1
   HISTORICAL BACKGROUND OF DR SEBI 1

DR SEBI DIET DO YOU REALLY NEED IT? THIS WILL HELP YOU DECIDE! 2
   INTRODUCTION TO DR SEBI DIET 2
      ALKALINE PLANT FOOD 2
      THE BODY SYSTEM PH MEASURE 3
      DR SEBI ALKALINE BASED DIET 3
   DR SEBI'S RECOMMENDED FOOD LIST 4
      FRUITS 4
      VEGETABLES 4
      OILS 4
      MILK 5
      GRAINS 5
      LEGUMES 5
      NUTS AND SEEDS 5
      SEASONINGS 5
      HERBAL TEAS 5

THE ULTIMATE NUTRITIONAL GUIDE TO DR SEBI'S DIET PLAN 6
   The Guideline Rules to Follow on Dr. Sebi diet 6
   THE MEAL PLAN: 30 DAYS TO A BETTER DR SEBI COOKBOOK 6
      WEEK 1 7
      WEEK 2 8
      WEEK 3 9
      WEEK 4 10

THE HIDDEN MYSTERY BEHIND DR SEBI'S RECIPES AND SUPPLEMENT REVEAL 11
   30 day to detox: INTRODUCTION TO FOOD RECIPES 11

"30 DAY TO DETOX" COOKBOOK: DR SEBI'S CELL FOOD RECIPES AND DIRECTIONS 13
   DAY 1 13
      BREAKFAST - BANOFFEE CRUMBLE 13
      LUNCH - AVOCADO SEEDS 13

 DINNER - CABBAGE ZUCCHINI SALAD 14

DAY 2 15
 BREAKFAST - CABBAGE DILL SALAD 15
 LUNCH - ELDERBERRY TEA 15
 DINNER - CUCUMBER ONION SALAD 16

DAY 3 17
 BREAKFAST - YUMMY CAULIFLOWER SOUP 17
 LUNCH - CREAMY CELERY SOUP 17
 DINNER - ALKALINE CORNBREAD 18

DAY 4 19
 BREAKFAST - CREAMY BROCCOLI SOUP 19
 LUNCH - CAESAR SALAD 19
 DINNER - KALE AVOCADO SALAD 20

DAY 5 21
 BREAKFAST - HEALTHY CINNAMON FLAX SEED PORRIDGE 21
 LUNCH - CREAMY CAULIFLOWER GREEN SOUP 21
 DINNER - HEALTHY GARLIC SPINACH 22

DAY 6 23
 BREAKFAST - BROCCOLI SPINACH COCONUT CURRY 23
 LUNCH - MUSHROOM GARLIC BOK CHOY 23
 DINNER - TASTY PUMPKIN SPICED SOUP 24

DAY 7 25
 BREAKFAST - CUCUMBER DRESSING 25
 LUNCH - MANGO CHIA SEED PUDDING 25
 DINNER - THE KIDNEY CLEANSE JUICE 26

DAY 8 27
 BREAKFAST - DR. SEBI'S FALL APPLE CRUMBLE 27
 LUNCH - DR. SEBI'S PORTOBELLO TACOS 27
 DINNER - WINTER GREENS KALE SALAD WITH CREAMY CITRUS VINAIGRETTE 28

DAY 9 30
 BREAKFAST - WHEY PROTEIN BLAST 30
 LUNCH - ROASTED SWISS CHARD AND POTATO CAKE 30

DINNER - ROASTED SQUASH WITH LEMON 31

DAY 10 32

BREAKFAST - TACOS WITH SWEET POTATO HASH 32

LUNCH - SUNRISE BREAKFAST SMOOTHIE 32

DINNER - SHRIMP AND MANGO CEVICHE 33

DAY 11 34

BREAKFAST - PEANUT BUTTER AND SMOOTHIE 34

LUNCH - BAKED MILLET AND APPLE BREAKFAST CAKES 34

DINNER - AMARANTH BANANA PORRIDGE 35

DAY 12 36

BREAKFAST - DR. SEBI'S CREAMY VEGETABLE SOUP 36

LUNCH - DR. SEBI'S TOASTED QUINOA SALAD 36

DINNER - DR. SEBI'S PORTOBELLO TACOS 37

DAY 13 38

BREAKFAST - POWERFUL HEALING SOUP 38

LUNCH - FALL-INSPIRED PEAR WALNUT SALAD 38

DINNER - THE AVOCADO, APPLE, AND WALNUT HUMMUS 39

DAY 14 40

BREAKFAST - DR. SEBI'S ORIGINAL "BROMIDE PLUS" SMOOTHIE 40

LUNCH - DR. SEBI'S PORTOBELLO MUSHROOM BURGERS 40

DINNER - DR. SEBI'S SLEEPY TIME DRINK 41

DAY 15 42

BREAKFAST - DR. SEBI'S BLUEBERRY SMOOTHIE 42

LUNCH - DR. SEBI'S FAT-FREE PEACH MUFFINS 42

DINNER - CHERRY TOMATO SALAD 43

DAY 16 44

BREAKFAST - DR. SEBI'S TRIPLE BERRY SMOOTHIE 44

LUNCH - DR. SEBI'S BASIL PESTO "ZOODLES" 44

DINNER - IRRESISTIBLE RED PEPPER HUMMUS 45

DAY 17 46

BREAKFAST - KAMUT PORRIDGE 46

LUNCH - DR. SEBI'S WATERMELON REFRESHER 46

DINNER - DR. SEBI'S HERBAL SMOOTHIE 47

DAY 18 48

BREAKFAST - DR. SEBI'S DETOX BERRY SMOOTHIE 48

LUNCH - DR. SEBI'S "HEART-FRIENDLY" SALSA 48

DINNER - DR. SEBI'S CLEANSING GREEN SOUP 49

DAY 19 50

BREAKFAST - BANANA NUT MUFFINS 50

LUNCH - DR. SEBI'S "BLISSFUL" SMOOTHIE 50

DINNER - ASIAN CUCUMBER SALAD 51

DAY 20 52

BREAKFAST - SCRUMPTIOUS MANGO "CHEESECAKE" 52

LUNCH - DR. SEBI'S "BRAIN-BOOSTING" SMOOTHIE 52

DINNER - ONE-POT ZUCCHINI MUSHROOM PASTA 53

DAY 21 54

BREAKFAST - DR. SEBI'S SEA MOSS PANNA COTTA 54

LUNCH - DR. SEBI'S HEAVY METAL DETOX SMOOTHIE 54

DINNER - DR. SEBI'S "OWL" BLUEBERRY PANCAKES 55

DAY 22 56

BREAKFAST - DR. SEBI'S FANTASTIC QUINOA BREAD 56

LUNCH - ALL-NATURAL TAMARIND PASTE 56

DINNER - DR. SEBI'S CREAMY VEGETABLE SOUP 57

DAY 23 58

BREAKFAST - HEALTHY "FRIED-RICE" 58

LUNCH - VEGGIE FAJITAS TACOS 58

DINNER - CLASSIC HOMEMADE HUMMUS 59

DAY 24 60

BREAKFAST - JUICY PORTOBELLO BURGERS 60

LUNCH - THE GRILLED ROMAINE LETTUCE SALAD 60

DINNER - WAKAME SALAD 61

DAY 25 62

BREAKFAST - BERRY SORBET 62

LUNCH - CHAMOMILE DELIGHT SMOOTHIE 62

DINNER - DR. SEBI'S ENERGIZER SMOOTHIE ... 62

DAY 26 ... 63
BREAKFAST - DR. SEBI'S ORANGE CREAMSICLE SMOOTHIE ... 63
LUNCH - STEWED OKRA AND TOMATOES ... 63
DINNER - DR. SEBI'S CHICKPEA LOAF ... 63

DAY 27 ... 65
BREAKFAST - MAGNESIUM-BOOSTING SMOOTHIE ... 65
LUNCH - ALKALINE-ELECTRIC CLASSIC APPLE BAKE ... 65
DINNER - PLANT-BASED QUINOA BOWL ... 65

DAY 28 ... 67
BREAKFAST - GREEN PANCAKES ... 67
LUNCH - DR. SEBI'S NO-BAKE ENERGY BALLS ... 67
DINNER - DR. SEBI'S MANGO SALAD ... 68

DAY 29 ... 69
BREAKFAST - PLANT-BASED CHICKPEA QUINOA BURGERS ... 69
LUNCH - ALKALINE-ELECTRIC ICE CREAM ... 69
DINNER - TEF GRAIN BURGERS ... 70

Day 30 ... 71
BREAKFAST - ALKALINE-ELECTRIC SPRING SALAD ... 71
LUNCH - IMMUNITY-BOOSTING SMOOTHIE ... 71
DINNER - PLANT-BASED MUSHROOM GRAVY! ... 72

DR SEBI'S CELL FOOD SUPPLEMENT ... 73
THE WHOLE FOOD SUPPLEMENT ... 73
WHAT SUPPLEMENTS SHOULD YOU TAKE? ... 73

MAINTENANCE PROGRAM: FOOD PLAN FOR WEIGHT MAINTENANCE ... 78
How to develop successful strategies for weight maintenance after weight loss? ... 78

CONCLUSIONS ... 81

ABOUT THE AUTHOR ... 82
BIOGRAPHY ... 82
Books By Elizabeth Bowman ... 83

DR. SEBI JOURNAL ... 84

30 DAYS TO DETOX AND IMPROVE YOURSELF. IN THIS MOTIVATION JOURNAL BASED ON DR. SEBI'S PLANT-BASED ALKALINE DIET, YOU CAN KEEP TRACK OF YOUR MEALS, GOALS, AND PROGRESS. *84*

NUTRITIONAL GUIDE 85

How to compile the "Detox Daily Diary" 86
Daily Diary Instructions 87
- *COUNTDOWN* *87*
- *SHOPPING LIST* *87*
- *MEAL PLANNER* *87*
- *VOTE* *87*
- *NOTES* *87*
- *WATER TRACKER* *87*
- *TO DO LIST* *87*
- *CITATIONS* *87*

Weekly Results Instructions 88
Monthly Results Instructions 88
HOW TO PRINT THE PLANNER 88
- *REMEMBER!* *142*

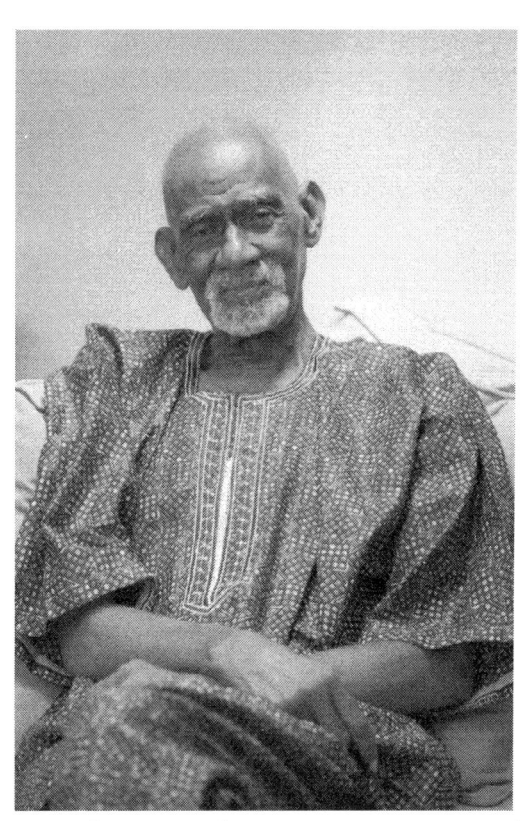

"You don't have to eat less. You just have to eat right."

Dr. Alfredo "Sebi" Bowman

INTRODUCTION

HISTORICAL BACKGROUND OF DR SEBI

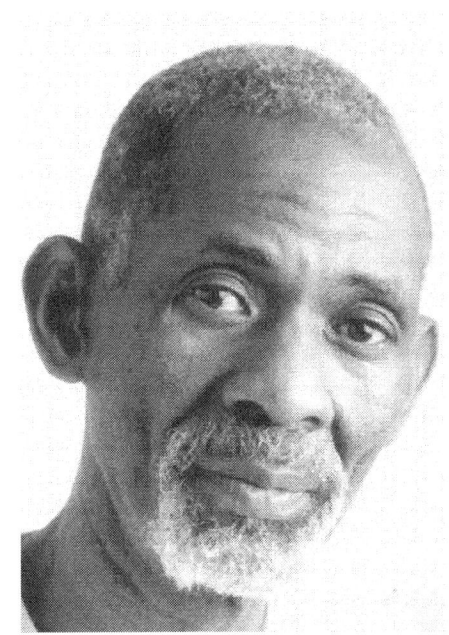

Alfredo Darrington Bowman, also known as Dr. Sebi, was a Honduran herbalist and self-proclaimed healer. He had a colorful life, and he was often accused of being a fraud. He was arrested many times for various reasons, including money laundering charges. He, through all of this, remained faithful to his beliefs about foods and an Alkaline diet. He amassed a huge following of believers throughout his life, and his diet and teachings are still popular to this day. Born in Ilanga, Honduras, on 26th November 1933, he died on the 6th August 2016, aged 82, while being held under arrest. Many people thought his death was not a coincidence and was part of a conspiracy to silence him as he was outspoken about conventional medicines and large drug companies.

As purists will know, Dr. Sebi would never recommend foods that are not on his specifically recommended foods list. These foods are known a Cell food. If you are looking to follow the Alkaline food lifestyle diet, you need to be aware of these recommended foods. This little book is designed to help you choose these foods. The Dr. Sebi food list is precise; however, it surprisingly doesn't contain many very popular plant-derived/based foods that many people recognize as super whole foods. One surprising food that does not appear in this list is garlic. Dr. Sebi regarded it as dangerous and avoided it at all costs. Dr. Sebi disapproved of hybrid foods, i.e., plant foods derived from unnatural cross-pollination of two or more different plants. These he regarded as genetically modified. The reasoning for this was he believed that hybrids altered the PH balance and the electrical composition, thus altering the genetic make-up to the detriment of the human body. Here is a list of Dr. Sebi approved foods recognized as suitable and safe for an Alkaline diet for the human body.

PART ONE

DR SEBI DIET DO YOU REALLY NEED IT? THIS WILL HELP YOU DECIDE!

INTRODUCTION TO DR SEBI DIET

ALKALINE PLANT FOOD

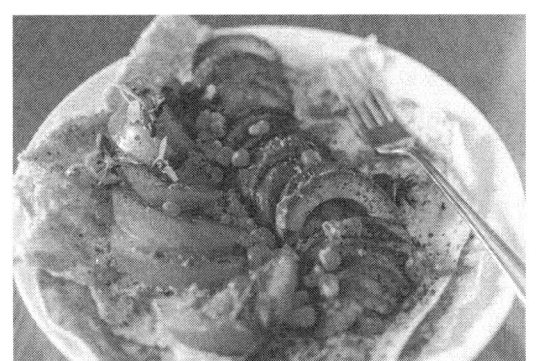

The globalized western diet, which centralized on processed food, dairy, and hybridized and genetically modified plant foods, needed to be avoided and changed to the consumption of natural alkaline plant foods. We must examine the plant foods indigenous to Africa or other areas of the world that share the same or similar environmental conditions of Africa, like Central and South America, the Caribbean, and India. These foods grow under the same conditions that supported and developed the African genome and supported and developed the plants' genome with chemical affinities with the African genome, which is the foundation of the human genome in all people.

Plants supported the health of the body system in two ways. First, they make available a wide array of minerals, vitamins, carbohydrates, fats, and protein in proportions that naturally supported the body's nutrients. The bodies can use the nutrients to replace the nutrients lost through metabolic processes that support organ function. Secondly, the bodies can use the plant's phytonutrients, specific, and various chemical compounds in plants, which the plants used to protect themselves against disease. The hospitable environment of Africa and similar environments abundantly and naturally produced plants that amply supplied both.

THE BODY SYSTEM PH MEASURE

In the early days of studies, we came across the terms "Acid and Alkaline" Acids and alkalis are substances found in nature. They determine on a pH scale that measures if they are acidic or alkaline, giving us an idea about their reactivity. On the scale, a pH of '0' is known as the most acidic, and a pH of '14' is accepted as the most alkaline. Water (H2O) has a pH of 7 and is believed to be neutral, while anything above 7 is alkaline.

The human body is a bit alkaline with a pH of about 7.4, while the stomach is acidic with a pH range of 2-3.5 for the breakdown of food particles. The pH of urine and saliva can vary depending on our eating and the medications' intake. But the pH of blood is slightly more alkaline with a pH value of 7.36-7.44, which can be used in determining the overall health or well-being of an individual.

DR SEBI ALKALINE BASED DIET

The Dr. Sebi alkaline diet, does the self-educated herbalist create a plant-based diet Alfredo Darrington Bowman claimed to rejuvenate the body cells by eliminating toxic waste through alkalizing the blood PH value. The diet claims to eat a shortlist of approved foods along with many supplements. He designed this diet for individuals who decided to naturally cure or prevent disease and improve their overall health without conventional Western medicine. He believes that diseases cannot operate in an alkaline system, but they exist when the body becomes too acidic. He claimed to restore the body's natural alkaline state by following his prescribed supplements and detoxify your diseased body.

The herbalist Dr. Sebi was pivotal in reestablishing the idea that alkaline nonhybrid plant foods had chemical affinities with the body and supported healing. His African Bio Mineral Balance methodology of recovery is based on the premise that food that raises the body's acidity level and causes mucus's overproduction in the body is the disease's root. Acidic and toxin-laden foods continuously attack the body, cause a prolonged inflammatory reaction, and lead to chronic inflammation.

An alkaline diet maintains the consumption of vegetables, herbal spices, fresh fruit juices, seeds and nuts by reducing sugary and processed food like caffeine, sweets, and alcohol. It is based on the meal that is replacing acid-forming foods with alkaline foods for health benefits in positive ways. The consumers and researchers of this diet claim that this diet can affect the body's pH value by taking more alkaline-based food, which is in line with the metabolic process. After food breakdown, metabolic particles remain in the body, which can be either acidic or alkaline, depending on the food items' nature. Acidic particles can cause damage to the body and make it vulnerable to diseases, while alkaline residue has a protective effect on the body.

Generally, diet components like protein, phosphate, and sulfur are accepted to leave an acidic residue, whereas calcium, magnesium, and potassium produce alkaline residue in the body. Alkaline diet alone is never a good deal because a healthy balance of the nutrition-specific diet is body requirements. This includes nutrition from protein sources, nuts, legumes, fresh vegetables and elimination of processed and packaged food items from your list. Dr. Sebi's recommendations lists of foods are the modified and healthy alkaline-based recipes.

DR SEBI'S RECOMMENDED FOOD LIST

The food list is divided into different categories such as:

FRUITS

Fruits are natural and are the body's natural and primary source of energy. Healthy to consume fresh fruits and not canned fruits, which are processed and contain cancer-causing additives and preservatives.

Recommended: **Apples, bananas, currants**, dates, figs, berries, cantaloupe, cherries, grapes (seeded), oranges, papayas, peaches, pears, plums key limes, mango, melons (seeded), soursops, tamarind prickly pear, prunes, raisins (seeded), soft jelly coconuts,.

VEGETABLES

Vegetables are high in micronutrients, including minerals, phytonutrients, vitamins, and fiber, which also serve to feed the body and cleanse the digestive system containing most of the body's immune system.

Recommended: Amaranth greens (callaloo), , sea vegetables (wakame, dulse, arame, hijiki, nori), squash, tomato (cherry and plum only), tomatillo, turnip greens, watercress, zucchini, avocado, bell peppers, chayote (Mexican squash), purslane (verdolaga), poke salad, cucumber, dandelion greens, Kale, lettuce (except iceberg), garbanzo beans (chickpeas), green banana, izote (cactus leaf), mushrooms (except shitake), nopales, okra, olives, onions,

OILS

It is better to minimize the use of oils because they are not whole food, and much oil usage can lead to inflammation, support the development of diabetes, and damage arteries.

Recommended: Grapeseed oil (minimize use because it is high in omega-6), sesame oil, hemp-seed oil, avocado oil, olive oil (better not to cook with – destroys the integrity of the oil at high heat), coconut oil (better not to cook with – destroys the integrity of the oil at high heat.)

MILK

Hemp-seed milk, coconut milk, walnut milk. (It is better to make your milk than to buy it to make sure you are drinking pure nut or seed milk).

GRAINS

Recommended: Amaranth, fonio, Kamut, quinoa, rye, spelled, teff, wild rice

LEGUMES

Recommended: Garbanzo beans (chickpeas)

NUTS AND SEEDS

Recommended: Brazil nuts, hemp seeds, pine nuts, raw sesame "tahini" butter, walnuts

SEASONINGS

Recommended: Achiote, basil, bay leaf, Cayenne (African bird pepper), cilantro, coriander, dill, habanero, onion powder, oregano, powdered granulated seaweed (kelp, dulce, nori), savory, sweet basil, tarragon, pure sea salt, sage, thyme.

HERBAL TEAS

Drinking herbal teas than regular teas is of greater health, such as green tea, because they don't have caffeine and contain a wide range of phytonutrients that support the immune system.

Recommended: Alvaca, anise, chamomile, cloves, fennel, ginger, lemongrass, red raspberry, sea-moss tea.

THE ULTIMATE NUTRITIONAL GUIDE TO DR SEBI'S DIET PLAN

THE GUIDELINE RULES TO FOLLOW ON DR. SEBI DIET

- You should never use any foods which are not listed.
- Do not use a Microwave cooker, any canned foods, or any seedless fruits.
- No Animal products, Meat, Fish, Dairy, Honey, White or Brown sugars, and no Alcohol.
- Drink as much Springwater as possible.
- Eat cell food before taking medicines, Sleep as much as possible, particularly during Detoxing.
- Take Dr. Sebi's supplement one hour before western medicine.

THE MEAL PLAN: 30 DAYS TO A BETTER DR SEBI COOKBOOK

Are you in search of a daily or monthly meal plan but can't seem to find highly effective ones that work for you? It's your lucky time! Look through the below recipes of a 30-day meal plan ideas concordant with Dr. Sebi's diet and recommendations. Meal planning is a great insight to enforce that you and your family maintain healthy eating habits. You will never run dry of dish ideas with this extensive collection of meal plans. The possibilities are endless! Let your creativity and cooking experience guide you. Your favorite 30day-long meal plan is right around the corner.

These sample meal plans focus on the approved ingredients included in the diet's nutritional guide by Dr. Sebi. Meals on this plan emphasize vegetables, spices, and fruits with small amounts of the other food groups.

WEEK 1

	DAYS	BREAKFAST	LUNCH	DINNER
1	MONDAY	Banoffee Crumble	Avocado seeds	Cabbage Zucchini Salad
2	TUESDAY	Cabbage Dill Salad	Elderberry tea	Cucumber Onion Salad
3	WEDNESDAY	Yummy Cauliflower Soup	Creamy Celery Soup	Alkaline Cornbread
4	THURSDAY	Creamy Broccoli Soup	Caesar Salad	Kale Avocado Salad
5	FRIDAY	Healthy Cinnamon Flax Seed Porridge	Creamy Cauliflower Green Soup	Healthy Garlic Spinach
6	SATURDAY	Broccoli Spinach Coconut Curry	Mushroom Garlic Bok Choy	Tasty Pumpkin Spiced Soup
7	SUNDAY	Cucumber Dressing	Mango Chia Seed Pudding	The Kidney Cleanse Juice

WEEK 2

	DAYS	BREAKFAST	LUNCH	DINNER
8	MONDAY	Dr. Sebi's Fall Apple Crumble	Dr. Sebi's Portobello Tacos	Winter Greens Kale Salad With Creamy Citrus Vinaigrette
9	TUESDAY	Whey Protein Blast	Roasted Swiss Chard and Potato Cake	Roasted Squash with Lemon
10	WEDNESDAY	Tacos with Sweet Potato Hash	Sunrise Breakfast Smoothie	Shrimp and Mango Ceviche
11	THURSDAY	Peanut Butter and Smoothie	Baked Millet and Apple Breakfast Cakes	Amaranth Banana Porridge
12	FRIDAY	Dr. Sebi's Creamy Vegetable Soup	Dr. Sebi's Toasted Quinoa Salad	Dr. Sebi's Portobello Tacos
13	SATURDAY	Powerful Healing Soup	Fall-inspired Pear Walnut Salad	The Avocado, Apple, and Walnut Hummus
14	SUNDAY	Dr. Sebi's Original "Bromide Plus" Smoothie	Dr. Sebi's Portobello Mushroom Burgers	Dr. Sebi's Sleepy Time Drink

WEEK 3

	DAYS	BREAKFAST	LUNCH	DINNER
15	MONDAY	Dr. Sebi's Blueberry Smoothie	Dr. Sebi's Fat-Free Peach Muffins	Cherry Tomato Salad
16	TUESDAY	Dr. Sebi's Triple Berry Smoothie	Dr. Sebi's Basil Pesto "Zoodles"	Irresistible Red Pepper Hummus
17	WEDNESDAY	Kamut Porridge	Dr. Sebi's Watermelon Refresher	Dr. Sebi's Herbal Smoothie
18	THURSDAY	Dr. Sebi's Detox Berry Smoothie	Dr. Sebi's "Heart-Friendly" Salsa	Dr. Sebi's Cleansing Green Soup
19	FRIDAY	Banana Nut Muffins	Dr. Sebi's "Blissful" Smoothie	Asian Cucumber Salad
20	SATURDAY	Scrumptious Mango "Cheesecake"	Dr. Sebi's "Brain-Boosting" Smoothie	One-Pot Zucchini Mushroom Pasta
21	SUNDAY	Dr. Sebi's Sea Moss Panna Cotta	Dr. Sebi's Heavy Metal Detox Smoothie	Dr. Sebi's "Owl" Blueberry Pancakes

WEEK 4

	DAYS	BREAKFAST	LUNCH	DINNER
22	MONDAY	Dr. Sebi's Fantastic Quinoa Bread	ALL-NATURAL Tamarind Paste	Dr. Sebi's Creamy Vegetable Soup
23	TUESDAY	Healthy "Fried-Rice"	Veggie Fajitas Tacos	Classic Homemade Hummus
24	WEDNESDAY	Juicy Portobello Burgers	The Grilled Romaine Lettuce Salad	Wakame Salad
25	THURSDAY	Berry Sorbet	Chamomile Delight Smoothie	Dr. Sebi's Energizer Smoothie
26	FRIDAY	Dr. Sebi's Orange Creamsicle Smoothie	Stewed Okra and Tomatoes	Dr. Sebi's Chickpea Loaf
27	SATURDAY	Magnesium-Boosting Smoothie	Alkaline-Electric Classic Apple Bake	Plant-Based Quinoa Bowl
28	SUNDAY	Green Pancakes	Dr. Sebi's No-Bake Energy Balls	Dr. Sebi's Mango Salad
29	MONDAY	Plant-Based Chickpea Quinoa Burgers	Alkaline-Electric Ice Cream	Tef Grain Burgers
30	TUESDAY	Alkaline-Electric Spring Salad	Immunity-Boosting Smoothie	Plant-based mushroom gravy

PART TWO

THE HIDDEN MYSTERY BEHIND DR SEBI'S RECIPES AND SUPPLEMENT REVEAL

30 DAY TO DETOX: INTRODUCTION TO FOOD RECIPES

"Everyone should be his own physician. We ought to assist and not force nature. Eat with moderation what agrees with your constitution. Nothing is excellent for the body but what we can process and digest. What medicine can produce digestion? Exercise. What will recruit strength? Sleep. What will alleviate incurable ills? Patience."

— Voltaire-

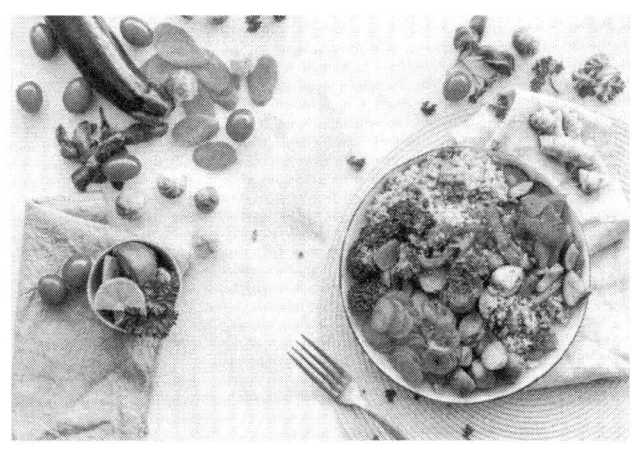

Everyone is baffled about what is right to eat nowadays. Several diets range from eating only plants to eating a diet primarily of animal foods — vegan, vegetarian, Mediterranean, Paleo, grain-free, raw food diet, and everything in between. Proponents of each diet proclaim that they know the ticket to health, justifying their points with well-documented research and case studies. For many, creating nourishing meals has become confusing and stressful rather than a joyous process.

Dr. Sebi food in particular; however, it surprisingly doesn't contain many very popular plant-derived/based foods that many people recognize as super whole foods. His food recommendations are specific foods recommended for sound health proven from research and studies. These foods are known as Cell food and are categorized into different sections. The Food which are divided under categories of Vegetables, Fruits, Herbal teas, Grains, Seeds &

Nuts, Oils and Spices & Seasonings, and food are sub-divided into Mild, Spicy, Salty and Sweet.

In the next chapter of the book, we will be discussing the recipes of a few selected food out of the list of approved food based on Dr. Sebi's nutritional guide.

"30 DAY TO DETOX" COOKBOOK: DR SEBI'S CELL FOOD RECIPES AND DIRECTIONS

DAY 1

BREAKFAST - BANOFFEE CRUMBLE

Ingredients:

For the filling
- 4-6 bananas, depending on size, sliced lengthways
- 397g tin of carnation caramel
- For the crumble
- 180g plain/all-purpose flour
- 90g unsalted butter, cubed
- 60g soft light brown sugar
- 1/4 tsp (or more if you desired!) grated nutmeg

Directions

1. Heat the oven to about 170C/340F.
2. Slice the bananas and place them at the bottom of baking dish
3. Spread the caramel over the bananas, pushing it down to create a smooth layer of caramel, make sure your bananas are completely covered.
4. Place all the rest of your ingredients into a large bowl.
5. Rub the butter between your fingertips to create the crumble mix, making sure no large lumps of butter are left.
6. Sprinkle crumbles mix over the fruit and caramel in the baking dish.
7. Place your dish in the oven for twenty minutes, until golden and beautiful, once out of the oven, then cool for 5 minutes before serving.

LUNCH - AVOCADO SEEDS

Special benefit

- Reduce inflammation and ease joint pain
- Optimal for digestive health
- Destroys cancer cells
- Banish Cravings and Shed Fat
- Get Radiant Glowing Skin

Direction:

- Wash and dry the seed, boil for 15minutes and let it steep for 10min. It has such a smooth taste, not bitter at all. It's healthy to take sweet avocado tea with the addition of nectar in the summer period to chill.

DINNER - CABBAGE ZUCCHINI SALAD

Total Time: 15 minutes

Serving Size: 10

Ingredients:

- One medium zucchini, spiralized
- One tsp stevia
- 1/3 cup vinegar of rice
- 3/4 bottle of olive oil
- 1 cup of almonds, sliced
- 1 cup shelled sunflower seed
- 1 lb of cabbage, shredded

Directions:

1. Chop and set aside spiralized zucchini into small pieces
2. In a large mixing bowl, combine cabbage, almonds, and sunflower seeds.
3. Stir in zucchini.
4. In a small bowl, mix oil, stevia, and vinegar. Whisk well and pour over vegetables.
5. Toss salad well and place in the refrigerator for 2 hours.
6. Serve and enjoy.

DAY 2

BREAKFAST - CABBAGE DILL SALAD

Serving Size: 6
Total Time: 25 minutes

Ingredients:

- 2 lbs red cabbage, shred
- 2 tbsp fresh dill, chopped
- One orange juice
- 1 tbsp red wine vinegar
- One cinnamon stick
- 4 1/4 oz butter
- 1/4 tsp black pepper
- 1 tsp salt

Directions:

1. Heat butter over medium heat in the pan.
2. Add shredded cabbage to the pan and cook for 10-15 minutes.
3. Season with pepper and salt.
4. Add orange juice, vinegar, and cinnamon. Stir well and simmer for 5 minutes.
5. Remove pan from heat.
6. Add dill and lemon zest.
7. Serve and enjoy.

LUNCH - ELDERBERRY TEA

Total Time: 15 minutes
Serving Size: 2

Ingredients:

- Filtered water
- 2 TBSP dried elderberries
- ¼ tsp cinnamon
- ½ tsp turmeric powder
- 1 tsp raw honey (optional)

Direction:

1. Put water and elderberries into a small saucepan.
2. Add turmeric and cinnamon.
3. Reduce the heat, then boil and simmer for about 15 minutes
4. Put off the heat and let it cool for about 5 minutes.
5. Finally, strain through a fine-mesh strainer and pour into individual mugs.
6. Stir in raw honey if using.

Note:

For an iced tea, pour into a mason jar and allow cooling, then refrigerating for up to 1 week. Serve over ice if desired.

DINNER - CUCUMBER ONION SALAD

Total Time: 10 minutes

Serving Size: 4

Ingredients:

- Two large cucumbers, sliced
- 4 tbsp white vinegar
- 1/4 cup sour cream
- One garlic clove, grated
- 1 tbsp dill, chopped
- 1/4 cup red onion, sliced
- Pepper and Salt

Directions:

1. Add all ingredients into the large bowl and mixed them until well combined.
2. Place salad bowl in the refrigerator for 30 minutes.
3. Serve chilled and enjoy.

DAY 3

BREAKFAST - YUMMY CAULIFLOWER SOUP

Total Time: 35 minutes
Serving Size: 4

Ingredients:

- 1/2 head cauliflower, diced
- One garlic clove, minced
- 16 oz vegetable broth
- One small diced onion
- 1/4 tbsp of olive oil
- 1/2 tsp of salt

Directions:

1. Heat the olive oil in a saucepan over medium heat.
2. Add onion and garlic in a saucepan and cook for 4 minutes.
3. Add cauliflower and broth. Stir well and bring to boil.
4. Cover pan with lid and simmer for 15 minutes.
5. Season with salt.
6. Using a blender to puree the soup until smooth and creamy.
7. Serve and enjoy.

LUNCH - CREAMY CELERY SOUP

Total Time: 40 minutes
Serving Size: 4

Ingredients:

- 6 large celery stalks, chopped
- 1 tbsp of lime juice
- 1 tsp of dried dill
- 2 cups of water
- 1 tsp bottle of olive oil
- 1 cup of coconut milk
- 1 sliced onion
- 1/2 tsp black pepper
- 1 tsp of salt.

Directions:

1. Heat olive oil in a saucepan over medium heat.
2. Add onion and sauté for 3-4 minutes.
3. Add celery and cook for 3 minutes.
4. Add water and salt and simmer for 30 minutes over medium heat.

5. Using a blender puree the soup until smooth
6. Simmer for 5 minutes
7. Season with lemon juice, pepper, and dill.
8. Serve hot and enjoy!

DINNER - ALKALINE CORNBREAD

Total Time: 45 minutes

Ingredient:

- 2c Chickpea flour
- 1c applesauce(you can peel & blend two apples into a puree)
- 1/2c Grape seed oil
- 1tbsp seasoning
- 1c Brazil nut milk
- Water as needed

Direction:

1. Mix all ingredients
2. Use your spring water to thin out
3. Oil pan with grapeseed oil and add batter
4. Bake for 30mins or until you can stick a toothpick in and it comes out clean with no batter on it

DAY 4

BREAKFAST - CREAMY BROCCOLI SOUP

Total Time: 25 minutes
Serving Size: 3

Ingredients:

- 4 cup broccoli florets
- 1/2 tsp ground nutmeg
- 1 small avocado, peel and sliced
- 2 cups vegetable broth

Directions:

1. Add broth into the pot and bring to simmer over medium-high heat.
2. Add broccoli into the pot and cook for 8 minutes or until tender.
3. Reduce heat to low and add avocado and nutmeg. Stir well, and cooks continue for 4 minutes.
4. Using a blender, puree the soup until smooth.
5. Serve and enjoy.

LUNCH - CAESAR SALAD

Total Time: 20 minutes
Serving Size: 4

Ingredients:

- 2 tsp Dijon mustard
- 1 tbsp capers
- 1 tbsp caper brine
- Three garlic cloves, minced
- 12 cups romaine lettuce, chopped
- 4 tbsp hemp seeds
- 2 tbsp water
- 3 tbsp fresh lemon juice
- One ripe avocado
- Pepper
- Salt

Directions:

1. Add avocado, pepper, salt, mustard, capers, caper brine, garlic, water, and lemon juice in a blender and blend until smooth.
2. Pour avocado mixture and hemp seeds into the large mixing bowl and mix well.
3. Add chopped romaine lettuce in a bowl and toss well.
4. Serve and enjoy.

DINNER - KALE AVOCADO SALAD

Total Time: 30 minutes

Serving Size: 2

Ingredients:

- 1 medium avocado, cut and peel into cubes
- 2 tbsp of pine nuts
- 2 tbsp bottle of olive oil
- 1/2 small orange juice
- 1/2 of lime juice
- 2 cups of kale chopped
- 1/4 tsp black pepper
- 1/2 tsp sea salt

Directions:

1. Pour 2-liter of heated water into the pot.
2. Add Kale and salt into the pot and heat for 10-20 minutes.
3. set aside a well drained cool kale.
4. Add pine nuts, Kale and avocado into the mixing bowl and toss well.
5. Season salad with salt and pepper.
6. Put in a small bowl, mix orange juice, oil and lime juice and pour over salad.
7. Serve and enjoy.

DAY 5

BREAKFAST - HEALTHY CINNAMON FLAX SEED PORRIDGE

Total Time: 10 minutes
Serving Size: 1

Ingredients:

- 1 cup water
- 4 tbsp coconut milk
- 4 tbsp flaxseed
- 1/8 tsp cinnamon

Directions:

1. Add all ingredients into the microwave-safe bowl and mix well.
2. Cook on high for 2 minutes.
3. Serve and enjoy.

LUNCH - CREAMY CAULIFLOWER GREEN SOUP

Total Time: 45 minutes
Serving Size: 4

Ingredients:

- 4 cups cauliflower florets, chopped
- 2 tbsp butter
- 1/2 cup coconut milk
- 2 cups of water
- 4 cups vegetable broth
- 1 tsp curry powder
- Four garlic cloves, minced
- One small onion, chopped
- 3 cups baby spinach, chopped
- One bunch chard, chopped

Directions:

1. Melt butter in the saucepan over medium heat.
2. Add onion and sauté until softened.
3. Add garlic and sauté for a minute.
4. Add curry powder and sauté for a minute.
5. Meanwhile, heat cauliflower and vegetable broth in a pot over medium heat.
6. Bring to simmer for 10 minutes.
7. Add water and chard and simmer for another 10 minutes.

8. Remove from heat and stir in coconut milk and add sautéed garlic, onion, and spices.
9. Using a blender, puree the soup until smooth.
10. Season soup with pepper and salt.
11. Serve and enjoy.

DINNER - HEALTHY GARLIC SPINACH

Total Time: 15 minutes

Serving Size: 2

Ingredients:

- One bunch fresh spinach, wash and dry
- Four garlic cloves, sliced
- 1 tbsp olive oil
- Pepper
- Salt

Directions:

1. Heat the oil in the pan over medium heat.
2. Add garlic and cook for about 5 minutes.
3. Add spinach and cook until wilted for about 2 minutes.
4. Season with pepper and salt.
5. Serve and enjoy.

DAY 6

BREAKFAST - BROCCOLI SPINACH COCONUT CURRY

Total Time: 40 minutes

Serving Size: 4

Ingredients:

- 1/2 cup coconut cream
- 1/4 onion, sliced
- 4 tbsp coconut oil
- 1/2 cup spinach
- 1 cup broccoli florets
- 1 tbsp red curry paste
- 2 tsp soy sauce
- 1 tsp ginger, minced
- 1 tsp garlic, minced

Directions:

1. Heat 2 tbsp coconut oil to a pan over medium-high heat.
2. Add onion and cook until softened.
3. Add garlic and sauté for some minutes.
4. Reduce heat to medium-low and add broccoli and stir everything well.
5. Once broccoli is cooked, then move vegetables to the other side of the pan.
6. Add curry paste and cook for a minute.
7. Add spinach and cook until wilted.
8. Add coconut cream, remaining oil, ginger, and soy sauce. Stir well and simmer for 5 minutes.
9. Serve and enjoy.

LUNCH - MUSHROOM GARLIC BOK CHOY

Total Time: 15 minutes

Serving Size: 2

Ingredients:

- 10 oz bok Choy, rinsed, drained, and chopped
- 4 oz mushrooms, sliced
- Three garlic cloves, minced
- 1 1/2 tbsp olive oil
- 1/4 tsp salt

Directions:

1. Heat oil in the pan over high heat.
2. Add garlic, mushroom, salt, and Bok Choy and sauté until Bok Choy wilted.

3. Remove from heat and serve immediately and enjoy.

DINNER - TASTY PUMPKIN SPICED SOUP

Total Time: 55 minutes
Serving Size: 4

Ingredients:

- 1 cup pumpkin puree
- 1/2 tsp ginger, minced
- Two garlic cloves, minced
- 1/4 onion, chopped
- 4 tbsp butter
- 1 1/2 cups vegetable broth
- 1/2 cup heavy cream
- One bay leaf
- 1/8 tsp nutmeg
- 1/4 tsp coriander
- 1/4 tsp cinnamon
- 1/2 tsp pepper
- 1/2 tsp salt

Directions:

1. Melt butter in a saucepan over -low heat.
2. Add ginger, garlic, and onion to the pan and sauté for 2-3 minutes.
3. Add spices and stir well and cook for 2 minutes.
4. Add broth and pumpkin puree and mix well. Bring to boil, then reduce heat to low and simmer for 20 minutes.
5. Using a blender, puree the soup until smooth, then simmer for another 20 minutes.
6. Remove the pan from heat and add heavy cream and stir well.
7. Serve and enjoy.

DAY 7

BREAKFAST - CUCUMBER DRESSING

Total Time: 20 minutes
Serving Size: 3

Ingredient

- Three meds. cucumbers, peeled
- Ten almonds, raw, unsalted
- Four tbs. pure olive oil
- 1/4 cup fresh lime juice
- 1/4 cup green onions, chopped fine
- 1/2 tsp. thyme
- 1/2 tsp. sea salt
- 1/4 tsp. dill
- 1-1/2 cup spring water
- Few sprigs of cilantro, chopped.

Direction:

1. Blend 10 almonds in spring water for 2 minutes with high speed
2. Strain and set liquid aside
3. Puree cucumbers in the blender with almonds
4. Add lime juice, olive oil, and remaining ingredients
5. Lightly blend, adding liquid, if needed
6. Pour over your salad and enjoy!

LUNCH - MANGO CHIA SEED PUDDING

Total Time: 25 minutes
Serving Size: 4

Ingredient

- 2 cups of coconut milk
- ½ cup of chia seeds
- One teaspoon of vanilla (powder or concentrate)
- ¼ teaspoon of cardamom
- One medium measured mango
- Three tablespoons of coconut nectar or two tablespoons of date glue

Instructions

1. Blend chia seeds with coconut milk, coconut nectar, vanilla, and cardamom in a bowl and refrigerate up to expedite.
2. Cut the mango up into pieces and puree in a blender.

3. Serve in like manner – combine or serve in layers!

DINNER - THE KIDNEY CLEANSE JUICE

Ingredients:

- 1-2 cups of soft-jelly coconut water
- 4 seeded cucumbers
- 2-3 key limes
- 1 bunch basil or sweet basil leaves
- 1/2 tsp. Bromide Plus Powder

Instructions:

1. Juice cucumbers, key limes and basil,. If you don't have a juicer, you can process them in a high-speed blender with the soft-jelly coconut water.
2. Serve juice in a tall glass and add the soft jelly coconut water and Bromide Plus Powder. Mix well and enjoy

DAY 8

BREAKFAST - DR. SEBI'S FALL APPLE CRUMBLE

Ingredients:

Spiced apple filling

- 5 organic Braeburn apples, peeled and cut into 1-inch pieces
- 2 tablespoons fresh spring water
- ¼ teaspoon ground cloves
- Pinch of sea salt
- 1 tablespoon date sugar

Topping:

- ½ cup of ground walnuts
- ⅓ cup of spelt flour
- ⅓ cup of amaranth flour
- ⅓ cup of crushed walnuts
- ⅓ cup of date sugar
- ⅓ cup of grape seed oil
- Heaping ¼ teaspoon sea salt
- 1 teaspoon spring water, if needed

Instructions:

1. Preheat the oven to 400 °F and grease an 8x8-inch baking dish.
2. Make the filling: Combine the apples, and water in a saucepan and simmer over very low heat, covered, stirring occasionally (making sure the apples don't burn on the bottom of the pan) for 15 minutes. Uncover, stir, and add the ground cloves, date sugar, and sea salt. The apples should be tender.
3. Make the topping: In a food processor, place the flour, walnuts, date sugar, grapeseed oil, and sea salt, and pulse until crumbly. Add the water if needed.
4. Scoop the apple filling into the baking dish and sprinkle with the topping. Bake for 18 to 22 minutes or until lightly crisp on top.

LUNCH - DR. SEBI'S PORTOBELLO TACOS

Ingredients:

- 2 extra-large portobello mushrooms
- 2 red bell peppers
- ½ a red onion
- 1 cup chopped cherry tomatoes
- 8 homemade kamut flour tortillas

- 1 key lime
- Sea salt and cayenne pepper, or any other approved seasonings, to taste
- ½ cup grapeseed oil
- Avocado (optional)

Instructions:

1. Preheat oven to 425F
2. Slice the portobellos into ½ inch thick wedges and slice bell pepper into ½ thick strips. Cut the onion into ½ inch thick rings or half-moons.
3. Brush both sides of mushrooms liberally with the grapeseed oil, then use the remaining on the red bell pepper, tomatoes and onion lightly. Sprinkle portobellos with sea salt, cayenne pepper, and any approved seasoning or spices of your choosing.
4. Roast 20 minutes or until portobellos are fork-tender.
5. When ready to serve, warm the tortillas, and divide the portobellos and vegetables.
6. Serve the portobello tacos with avocado and key lime.

DINNER - WINTER GREENS KALE SALAD WITH CREAMY CITRUS VINAIGRETTE

Serves: 4

Ingredients:

For The Salad:

- 2 cups Kale (+ salt & oil for massaging)
- ½ cup Broccoli Slaw
- ½ cup Beet Greens
- ¼ cup Red Cabbage
- ½ cup Garbanzo Beans
- 2 tbsp. Roasted Walnuts
- 2 tbsp. Dried Cranberries
- 2 tbsp. Hemp Hearts
- 2 Morning Star Farms Buffalo Chik Patties, sliced (optional)

The Dressing:

- ½ cup Avocado Oil
- Juice of 1 Lemon
- Juice of 1 Orange
- Zest of ½ Orange
- 2 tbsp. Apple Cider Vinegar
- 1 tsp. Dijon Mustard

- 1 tbsp. Agave Nectar (or Honey)
- 1 clove Garlic, minced

Instructions

1. Prepare all vegetables, as needed. I recommend gently massaging the Kale prior to chopping (this will make it softer and easier to eat. Simply massage with oil and salt for a few minutes prior to cutting). Chop the other greens according to your personal size preference and place in a large mixing bowl.

2. Prepare the dressing in a sealable container. Shake vigorously prior to serving. (I use leftover condiment or pasta jars).

3. Add remaining ingredients and gently toss with the desired amount of dressing.

4. Serve with the desired protein. We used Morning Star Farms Buffalo Chick Patties (I love the spicy addition), but regular chicken or tofu would also go nicely.

5. Enjoy immediately. If preparing in advance, do not add the dressing until you're ready to consume.

DAY 9

BREAKFAST - WHEY PROTEIN BLAST

Serves: 1

Ingredients

- ¾ C. Frozen Blueberries
- ½ Banana
- 3 Tbsp. Protein Powder
- ½ C. Milk
- 2 Tsp. Honey
- 3 Ice Cubes
- 1 Tbsp. Ground Flaxseed

Directions

- Place everything into a blender, and pulse until smooth.

LUNCH - ROASTED SWISS CHARD AND POTATO CAKE

Serves: 8

Ingredients:

- 1 Tbsp. Butter
- 1 Tbsp. Extra Virgin Olive Oil
- 3 Cloves Garlic, Minced
- ½ Yellow Onion, Minced
- 3 Medium Potatoes, Sliced Thinly
- Salt and Pepper
- 1 Bunch Swiss Chard, Chopped
- 1 C. Grated Jarlsberg Cheese

Directions:

1. Preheat the oven to 350 degrees Fahrenheit. Heat the oil and butter together in a ten-inch cast-iron skillet.
2. Sauté the onions and garlic until the onions are translucent, around five minutes. Spread the onions in the bottom of the skillet, and remove it from the heat.
3. Spread out a third of the potatoes in a single layer

over the onions and season with pepper and salt.

4. Top with a third of the chard, and sprinkle a third of the cheese over the top. Repeat until you end with the cheese a third time.
5. Cover tightly with a piece of oiled foil and bake for an hour and fifteen minutes. Remove the foil, and then return the skillet to the oven and bake until the cheese begins to bubble, around fifteen more minutes.
6. Set it aside to rest, and slice into wedges to serve.

DINNER - ROASTED SQUASH WITH LEMON

Total Time: 1 hour 10 minutes

Serving Size: 3

Ingredients:

- 2 lbs summer squash, cut into 1-inch pieces
- 1 large lemon
- 1/8 tsp paprika
- 1/8 tsp pepper
- 1/8 tsp garlic powder
- 3 tbsp olive oil
- Pepper
- Salt

Directions:

1. Preheat the oven to 400 F.
2. Spray a baking tray with cooking spray.
3. Place squash pieces onto the prepared baking tray and drizzle with olive oil.
4. Season with paprika, pepper, and garlic powder.
5. Squeeze lemon juice over the squash and bake in a preheated oven for 50-60 minutes.
6. Serve immediately and enjoy.

DAY 10

BREAKFAST - TACOS WITH SWEET POTATO HASH

Serves: 4

Ingredients:

- ¼ C. Tomato Paste
- Juice Of 1 Lemon
- 2 Tbsp. Honey
- 1 Tbsp. Tamari
- 1 Tbsp. Paprika
- 1 Tsp. Ground Cumin
- ¼ Tsp Pepper
- 2 Small Sweet Potatoes, Diced
- 1 Yellow Bell Pepper, Diced
- 1 Red Bell Pepper, Diced
- ½ C. Diced Onion
- 3 Garlic Cloves, Sliced
- ½ C. Cilantro, Chopped
- Corn Tortillas, Warmed
- Salsa
- Sliced Avocado
- Hot Sauce

Directions:

1. Preheat your oven to 400 degrees. In a bowl, whisk the tomato paste through the pepper together.
2. Add the potatoes through the garlic and toss.
3. Spread onto a baking sheet that's been lined with parchment paper. Roast until the potatoes are tender and browned, around forty-five minutes.
4. Transfer the vegetables to a bowl and stir in the cilantro. Serve with the remainder of the ingredients.

LUNCH - SUNRISE BREAKFAST SMOOTHIE

Serves: 2

Ingredients:

- 1 Small Banana, Peeled
- 1 Small Carrot, Shredded
- ¾ C. Raspberries
- ½ C. Plain Yogurt
- ½ C. Unsweetened Vanilla Almond Milk
- ½ Medium Orange, Peeled
- ¼ C. Rolled Oats

Directions:

1. Combine everything in a blender, and pulse until smooth.
2. Enjoy.

DINNER - SHRIMP AND MANGO CEVICHE

Serves: 6-8

Ingredients:

- ¾ Lb. Peeled-and-Deveined Shrimp
- ½ C. Minced Red Onion
- 6 Tbsp. Lime Juice
- ¼ C. Cilantro, Chopped
- 1 Mango, Diced
- 1 Tomato, Diced
- 1 Jalapeño Peppers, Minced
- ¾ Tsp. Sea Salt

Directions:

1. Boil salted water, and cook the shrimp for one to two minutes.
2. Drain and rinse the shrimp under cool water.
3. Chop the shrimp into half-inch pieces, and put in a bowl.
4. Add the rest of the ingredients, and chill for an hour.

DAY 11

BREAKFAST - PEANUT BUTTER AND SMOOTHIE

Serves: 2

Ingredients:

- 2 C. Milk
- ¾ C. Plain Yogurt
- 2 Tbsp. Creamy Peanut Butter
- 6 Dates, Pitted and Chopped
- 1 Tbsp. Rose Water
- 2 Tsp. Flaxseed Oil
- ¼ Tsp. Ground Cardamom

Directions:

1. Put all in a blender and pulse until smooth.
2. Pour into two glasses, and enjoy.

LUNCH - BAKED MILLET AND APPLE BREAKFAST CAKES

Serves: 12

Ingredients:

- Canola Spray Oil
- 2 Apples, Grated
- 1 C. Uncooked Millet
- ¾ C. Raisins
- ½ C. Sunflower Seeds
- 5 Tbsp. Lemon Juice and It's Zest
- ¾ C. Apple Juice

Directions:

1. Preheat the oven to 350 degrees Fahrenheit. Spray a muffin tin with oil. In a bowl, stir the apples through the zest together. Place into the prepared pan and spoon a third of a cup of the mixture into every muffin tin.
2. Drizzle a tablespoon of apple juice over each muffin, and cover with foil. Bake for half an hour.
3. Uncover and bake for twenty minutes or until they're golden brown. Cool for half an hour.

DINNER - AMARANTH BANANA PORRIDGE

Serves: 6-8

Ingredients:

- 2 C. Amaranth
- 2 Cinnamon Sticks
- 4 Bananas, Diced
- 2 Tbsp. Chopped Pecans

Directions:

1. Combine the amaranth with four cups of water and the cinnamon sticks in a pot.
2. Add the banana and cover. Simmer around twenty-five minutes.
3. Remove and discard the cinnamon. Places into bowls, and top with pecans as a garnish.

DAY 12

BREAKFAST - DR. SEBI'S CREAMY VEGETABLE SOUP

Ingredients:

- One tablespoon grapeseed oil
- 1/4 of a yellow onion
- One bell pepper (red)
- One zucchini
- Cayenne pepper, to taste
- Sea salt, to taste
- Approved herbs (optional)
- 1 cup homemade walnut milk

Instructions:

1. Placed chopped onion in the grapeseed oil, then put in a pot.
2. Mix zucchin with chopped pepper together, then cook for 5 minutes.
3. Blend the soft vegetable with homemade walnut milk.
4. Simmer for 15 minutes. Season to taste.
5. Serve with fresh approved herbs

LUNCH - DR. SEBI'S TOASTED QUINOA SALAD

Ingredients:

- 2 ½ cups vegetable homemade broth
- Two teaspoons sea salt
- 2 cups quinoa
- Two green bell peppers halved lengthwise
- Red bell pepper, cored and diced
- Zucchini, cut into bite-sized chunks
- Two tablespoons grapeseed oil
- Sea salt and one avocado
- 3 cups wild arugula
- Red onion, to taste

Instructions:

1. Start heating the oven to 400 degrees.
2. Bring broth and salt to a simmer over medium heat and stir in the quinoa. Stir well, bring the quinoa to a low simmer, then low the heat and cover.
3. Off the heat after allowing to simmer for 20 minutes
4. Fluff the quinoa with a fork just before serving.

5. While quinoa is simmering, add bell peppers and zucchini to a sheet pan and toss with olive oil and sea salt to taste.

6. Roast in the oven for 10-12 minutes until everything is golden and tender.

7. Toss together, then garnish with onion and avocado as you fold in the quinoa. Enjoy your quinoa salad!

DINNER - DR. SEBI'S PORTOBELLO TACOS

Ingredients:

- Two extra-large portobello mushrooms
- Two red bell peppers
- ½ a red onion
- 1 cup chopped cherry tomatoes
- Eight homemade Kamut flour tortillas
- One key lime
- Sea salt and cayenne pepper, or any other approved seasonings, to taste
- ½ cup grapeseed oil
- Avocado (optional)

Instructions:

1. Heat the oven 425F

2. Cut bell pepper into ½ thick strips and the portobellos into ½ inch thick wedges

3. Slice the onion into ½ inch thick rings

4. Brush both sides of mushrooms liberally with the grapeseed oil, then use the remaining tomatoes, onion lightly, and red bell pepper. Sprinkle portobellos with sea salt, cayenne pepper, and any approved seasoning or spices of your choosing.

5. Roast 20 minutes or until portobellos are fork-tender.

6. When ready to serve, warm the tortillas, and divide the portobellos and vegetables.

7. Serve the portobello tacos with avocado and key lime.

DAY 13

BREAKFAST - POWERFUL HEALING SOUP

Powerful recipes you can take during fasting or detoxifying.

Ingredients:

- One handful of approved sea vegetables
- One handful of approved greens (wild arugula, lettuce, purslane, verdolaga)
- 1 cup of dandelion greens
- 1 cup of mushrooms (except shiitake)
- 1/4 cup of your preferred approved herbs

Instructions:

1. Simmer the detoxifying ingredients for 1 to 2 hours over a low flame.
2. Strain to drink as a broth, or if you prefer, leave the cut vegetables intact and enjoy a bowl.

LUNCH - FALL-INSPIRED PEAR WALNUT SALAD

Ingredients:

- 1/2 cup walnut halves
- 1/4 cup of agave syrup
- Small pinch of sea salt
- Eight big handfuls of wild arugula
- Two large pears
- Four tablespoons of olive oil
- 1/4 cup of key lime juice

Instructions:

1. Preheat oven to 350 °F (175 °C). Mix walnuts with one table spoon of agave syrup and a pinch of sea salt. Spread out on a lined baking tray and bake for 7 to 8 minutes until golden. Remove from the oven and set aside to cool.
2. Add the rest of the agave syrup, the key lime juice, the olive oil, and a pinch of the sea salt to a small jar. Put the lid on and shake well.
3. Wash the pears gently and halve them lengthways. Remove the cores with a teaspoon, then cut each half into long thin slices.
4. Add the arugula and sliced pear to a large salad bowl. Sprinkle over the

cooled walnuts and drizzle generously with the dressing just before serving.

DINNER - THE AVOCADO, APPLE, AND WALNUT HUMMUS

Serving: 4

Ingredients:

- 3.5 oz (100g) dried garbanzo beans
- One large ripe avocado
- Two tablespoons tahini (ground sesame seeds)
- Two or small onions, finely chopped
- Two key limes, juiced
- ½ teaspoon of sea salt
- 1.5 fl oz (50m)l spring water
- Pinch of Cayenne or African bird pepper
- ¼ apple, diced
- Four walnuts
- One cucumber, sliced diagonally (or any approved veggie you'd like to dip!)

Preparation:

- Soak dry garbanzo beans overnight (12 hours) in spring water. Alternatively, unsoaked beans can be cooked in a pressure cooker (45 minutes).

Direction:

1. Cook soaked garbanzo beans in a pan of boiling water (medium heat, 30 minutes) until soft.
2. Blend cooked garbanzo, avocado, tahini, onion, lime, salt, and water (slowly add more water as needed).
3. Sprinkle chopped apple, walnuts, and a pinch of cayenne pepper and serve with sliced cucumber.

DAY 14

BREAKFAST - DR. SEBI'S ORIGINAL "BROMIDE PLUS" SMOOTHIE

Ingredients:

- 1/2 tablespoon Bromide Plus Powder
- 1/4 cup agave syrup
- 1 cup fresh (approved) fruit
- 1-quart of boiling spring water
- Three tablespoons walnuts

Instructions:

1. To prepare Dr. Sebi's Original Bromide Plus Smoothie, combine agave syrup, fruit, walnuts, and Bromide Plus Powder in a high-speed blender.
2. Slowly add the quart of spring water, and blend for 3-4 minutes.
3. Let cool, and enjoy!

LUNCH - DR. SEBI'S PORTOBELLO MUSHROOM BURGERS

Ingredients:

- Six large portobello mushroom caps
- 4 tbsp avocado oil
- 2 tbsp agave syrup
- 2 tbsp key lime juice
- Extra veggies: bell peppers, onions, mushrooms, etc.
- Add sea salt and Cayenne pepper to taste

Instructions:

1. To prepare Dr. Sebi's Portobello Mushroom Burgers, begin by mixing the marinade ingredients into a small bowl.
2. Place the mushroom caps cap side down in a 9x13 baking dish and pour the marinade over the top. Let the mushrooms soak in the marinade for about 30 minutes, occasionally brushing the mushrooms' tops.
3. Grill mushrooms for 5-7 minutes per side, beginning with cap side down. Continue to brush the mushrooms with the marinade while they are cooking.

4. Serve on toasted (approved-grain) bread with your favorite toppings or with mixed vegetables.

DINNER - DR. SEBI'S SLEEPY TIME DRINK

Ingredients:

- 1/4 cup cooked quinoa
- 2 cups amaranth greens
- 1/2 cup Dr. Sebi's Nerve/Stress Relief Herbal Tea
- 1/2 cup Dr. Sebi's Stomach Relief Herbal Tea
- 1 burro banana
- 1/4 cup cherries
- Agave syrup, to taste

Instructions:

1. To prepare Dr. Sebi's Sleepy Time drink, start by brewing the tea according to instructions. Let cool.
2. Blend all the ingredients in a high-speed blender and enjoy

DAY 15

BREAKFAST - DR. SEBI'S BLUEBERRY SMOOTHIE

Enjoy this delicious, nutritious blueberry smoothie as a snack or for breakfast! It will keep you energized and refreshed.

Ingredients:

- 1/4 cup cooked quinoa
- 1/2 cup blueberries
- 1 cup homemade walnut milk
- One burro banana
- 2 tbsp. date sugar

Instructions:

- Blend all ingredients in a high-speed blender and enjoy!

LUNCH - DR. SEBI'S FAT-FREE PEACH MUFFINS

Are you worried about your gallbladder health? Eating a low-fat diet can help manage and reduce gallstone symptoms. This recipe for Dr. Sebi's Fat-Free Muffins, is delicious, fat-free, and packed with good-for-you ingredients.

Ingredients:

- One tablespoon agave syrup
- Two large peaches about 2 cups, chopped
- 1 1/2 teaspoon mashed burro banana
- Two tablespoons warm spring water
- Two teaspoons key lime juice
- 1 1/4 cups homemade walnut milk
- 2 cups spelled flour
- 1/4 teaspoon salt
- 1/2 cup date sugar
- Two tablespoons chopped walnuts

Instructions:

1. Peel the peaches (if they are very ripe, the skin may easily peel off; if not, dip them in boiling water for 30 seconds and allow to cool before peeling) and remove the pit.
2. Chop into 1/2-inch pieces. Mix with agave syrup (optional) and set aside.
3. Add the key lime juice and walnut milk to the mashed burro banana and combine well.

4. Put in a large bowl, combine the flour, date sugar, and sea salt then mix well.

5. Add the liquid ingredients and stir just until combined; the batter will be thick. Fold in the peaches, making sure they are distributed throughout the batter.

6. Fill each muffin cup to within 1/2-inch of the top. Smooth the top of each muffin and, if desired, sprinkle with chopped walnuts.

7. Bake until a toothpick comes out clean, about 15-20 minutes. Allow the muffins to cool before serving. May easily peel off; if not, dip them in boiling.

DINNER - CHERRY TOMATO SALAD

Ingredients:

- 4 cups cherry tomatoes
- 1/4 cup red onion, chopped
- 1/4 cup fresh (approved) herbs such as dill, sweet basil, or thyme
- 1/4 cup olive oil
- 1 1/2 tablespoons key lime juice
- 1/4 teaspoon date sugar
- Salt and Cayenne pepper, to taste

Instructions:

1. To prepare your cherry tomato salad, start by placing the tomatoes, red onion, and herbs in a large bowl.

2. Now, let's make the dressing! In a small bowl, whisk together the olive oil, key lime juice, date sugar, sea salt, and cayenne pepper to taste.

3. Pour the dressing over the tomato mixture and gently toss to coat evenly. Serve, and enjoy!

DAY 16

BREAKFAST - DR. SEBI'S TRIPLE BERRY SMOOTHIE

People who eat diets high in fruits and vegetables have lower cancer rates, and berries may be among the most potent cancer-fighting fruits. Get all the power of berries with Dr. Sebi's Triple Berry Smoothie!

Ingredients:

- 1/2 cup strawberries
- 1/2 cup raspberries
- 1/2 cup blueberries
- 1 cup of water
- One burro banana
- Agave syrup, to taste

Instructions:

- Blend all ingredients in a high-speed blender and enjoy!

LUNCH - DR. SEBI'S BASIL PESTO "ZOODLES"

Fresh zucchini noodles tossed with basil pesto and cherry tomatoes make a light, healthy meal. Make this recipe for lunch or dinner, or serve it as a side!

Ingredients:

- 1 lb zucchini, in small strips
- 1 tbsp grapeseed oil
- One ripe avocado
- 1/2 cup packed basil leaves
- 1/4 cup walnuts
- 1/4 cup olive oil
- 1/2 teaspoon sea salt
- 1/4 teaspoon Cayenne pepper
- 1 cup cherry tomatoes
- juice of one key lime

Instructions:

1. To prepare your zoodles, begin by sauteing zucchini noodles with grapeseed oil until slightly tender but still crunchy.
2. Combine the remaining ingredients in a food processor or blender, and process into a creamy, thick paste.

3. Add to the drained pasta and toss and combine. If you find the sauce too thick, add a little bit of water.

4. Serve with cherry tomatoes halves and decorate with shredded dissected coconut as "cheese."

DINNER - IRRESISTIBLE RED PEPPER HUMMUS

Ingredients:

- 1 cup cooked chickpeas (garbanzo beans)
- Two tablespoons key lime juice
- Three tablespoons homemade tahini
- Two tablespoons olive oil
- One red bell pepper
- Sea salt and Cayenne pepper, to taste

Instructions:

1. Place the red bell pepper on the stove broiler and roast until the skin has become charred. Remove from fire and place in a plastic bag and wait for 10-15 minutes until they are cool enough to handle; then, remove the skin.

2. In the bowl of a food processor, combine the tahini and lime juice and process for 1 minute, scrape the sides and bottom of the bowl, then process for 30 seconds more. This extra time helps "whip" or "cream" the tahini, making the hummus smooth and creamy.

3. Add the olive oil, chickpeas, sea salt, and cayenne pepper. Process for 30 seconds, scrape the sides and bottom of the bowl, then process another 30 seconds or until well blended.

DAY 17

BREAKFAST - KAMUT PORRIDGE

Ingredients:

- 1 cup (7 ounces) Kamut
- 3 3/4 cups homemade walnut milk or soft-jelly coconut milk
- 1/2 teaspoon sea salt
- One tablespoon coconut oil
- Four tablespoons agave syrup

Instructions:

1. On a high-speed blender or food processor, mill the Kamut until you have about 1 1/4 cups of cracked Kamut.
2. In a medium saucepan, combine cracked Kamut, walnut or coconut milk, and sea salt and stir to combine.
3. Bring to a boil over high heat, then reduce heat to medium-low and simmer, occasionally stirring, until thickened to your liking, about 10 minutes.
4. Remove from heat, then stir in coconut oil and agave syrup. Garnish with fresh fruit if desired, and enjoy your Kamut porridge!

LUNCH - DR. SEBI'S WATERMELON REFRESHER

Ingredients:

- 4 cups cubed watermelon
- 2 cups soft-jelly coconut water
- Date sugar, to taste
- Zest and juice of 1 key lime

Instructions:

1. Place the watermelon and key lime juice and zest on a blender or food processor and blend until smooth.
2. Sweeten the mixture to taste with the date sugar. Keep in mind that the flavor will be watered down once you add the soft-jelly coconut water.
3. On a tall glass, serve 2/3 watermelon mixture and 1/3 soft-jelly coconut water. Mix with a spoon, and enjoy your Watermelon Refresher!

DINNER - DR. SEBI'S HERBAL SMOOTHIE

Ingredients:

- One tablespoon walnuts
- One burro banana
- One tablespoon date sugar or agave syrup

Instructions:

1. To make Dr. Sebi's Herbal Smoothie, start by preparing your Dr. Sebi's Herbal Tea according to the package instructions. Let cool.
2. Blend the tea with the walnuts, burro banana, and date sugar or agave syrup in a high-speed blender.
3. Enjoy!

DAY 18

BREAKFAST - DR. SEBI'S DETOX BERRY SMOOTHIE

Ingredients:

- One medium burro banana
- 1 Seville orange
- 1 cup berries (can be just blueberries or a mixture of blueberries, strawberries, and raspberries)
- 2 cups fresh lettuce
- One tablespoon hemp seeds
- Water
- 1/4 avocado, pitted

Instructions:

1. Add the water to your blender first, followed by the fruit and the greens.
2. Blend all ingredients until smooth and enjoy!

LUNCH - DR. SEBI'S "HEART-FRIENDLY" SALSA

Ingredients:

- 1 cup fresh blueberries
- 5 medium strawberries
- 1 pinch sea salt
- 2 tbsp. Grape seed oil
- 1/4 red onion
- 1/3 cup chopped green bell pepper
- 1/2 avocado, chopped
- Juice of two key limes

Instructions:

1. Combine blueberries, strawberries, onion, key lime zest, key lime juice, and green bell pepper in a food processor or blender and pulse about 5-6 times.
2. Taste and season with sea salt and cayenne pepper if desired.
3. Scrape salsa into a bowl and fold in chopped avocado.

DINNER - DR. SEBI'S CLEANSING GREEN SOUP

Serving: 4 plates

Ingredients:

- Three medium or two large yellow onions, peeled and roughly chopped
- One zucchini, washed but not peeled, and roughly chopped
- One bunch of dandelion greens
- One bunch wild arugula
- 4 cups homemade vegetable broth (made with approved vegetables only)
- 1/2 cup packed basil
- 1/2 cup packed dill
- Juice of 1 key lime
- Three tablespoons grapeseed oil
- 1/4 teaspoon sea salt
- 1/4 avocado
- Cayenne pepper, to taste

Instructions:

1. To make the cleansing soup, start by heating grapeseed oil in a large pot over medium-high until warm.
2. Add onions and cook for 5 minutes, occasionally stirring, until translucent.
3. Add dandelion greens, zucchini, and wild arugula, and cook for an additional 5 minutes.
4. Pour in homemade vegetable stock and bring to boil, then reduce heat to low and simmer, covered, for 15-20 minutes.
5. Let cool, uncovered, for 15 minutes.
6. If necessary, working in batches, blend with basil, avocado, dill, key lime juice, sea salt, and cayenne pepper until very smooth.
7. Serve and adjust seasonings. Decorate with fresh herbs.

DAY 19

BREAKFAST - BANANA NUT MUFFINS

Ingredients:

- 1 1/2 cups approved-flour
- 3/4 cup date sugar
- 1/2 teaspoon sea salt
- Two medium ripe burro bananas, mashed
- 3/4 cup homemade walnut milk
- 1/4 cup grapeseed oil
- One tablespoon key lime juice
- One medium ripe burro banana, cut into chunks
- 1/2 cup chopped walnuts, plus extra for sprinkling on top

Instructions:

- To prepare your Banana Nut Muffins, begin by preheating your oven to 400F (200C). Lightly grease the cups of a muffin pan or fill with 12 nonstick liners.

1. In a large bowl, mix all of the dry ingredients.
2. In a medium bowl, mix mashed banana with all of the wet ingredients. Add the wet into dry, and mix until it's just starting to come together. Be careful not to over mix. Add in the chopped banana and walnuts and give it 3 to 4 more stirs.
3. Divide the batter evenly among the muffin pan and finish by sprinkling extra walnuts on top (optional). Bake for 22 to 26 minutes until the muffins have risen and are golden brown on the edges, and a toothpick inserted into the center of a muffin comes out clean. Let cool for at least 10 minutes before enjoying.

LUNCH - DR. SEBI'S "BLISSFUL" SMOOTHIE

Ingredients:

- One pear, chopped
- 1/4 avocado, pitted
- 1 oz. blueberries
- 1/4 cup cooked quinoa
- 1 cup of water

Instructions:

- To prepare your smoothie, blend all ingredients in a high-speed blender and enjoy!

DINNER - ASIAN CUCUMBER SALAD

Ingredients:

- Three tbs. key lime juice
- One tbs. sesame oil
- 1/2 tsp. date sugar
- 1/4 tsp. sea salt
- One tbs. grated ginger
- One tbs. sesame seeds
- One tbs. powdered granulated seaweed

Instructions:

- To prepare your Asian Cucumber Salad, just toss everything together and enjoy!

DAY 20

BREAKFAST - SCRUMPTIOUS MANGO "CHEESECAKE"

Ingredients:

Crust:
- 1 cup walnuts
- 1/4 cup shredded dissected soft-jelly coconut
- 1 cup dates

Filling:
- 2 cups walnuts, soaked overnight & drained
- 1 cup homemade soft-jelly coconut milk
- 1/3 cup agave
- Juice of 1 key lime
- 1 tbsp. key lime zest
- Two large mangos, peeled and cut into cubes
- 6 tbsp. coconut oil

Instructions:

1. To prepare your plant-based mango "cheesecake," begin by lining an 8x8 inch baking sheet with parchment paper. Set aside.
2. In a food processor or high-speed blender, blend the walnuts, dates, and shredded soft-jelly coconut until combined. If your dough is not sticky enough, add a few more dates. Press the dough evenly into the bottom of your pan and place it in the freezer.
3. In a food processor or high-speed blender, add the walnuts and coconut milk. Blend until completely smooth, about 2-3 minutes. Next, add the coconut oil, agave syrup, key lime juice and zest, and mango cubes. Blend until combined.
4. Pour the cheesecake mixture into your pan, spreading evenly.
5. Place in the freezer to firm up 2-4 hours before serving. Serve frozen, or allow to thaw for 10-15 minutes for a softer texture.

LUNCH - DR. SEBI'S "BRAIN-BOOSTING" SMOOTHIE

Ingredients:

- 1 cup of Dr. Sebi's Nerve/Stress Relief Herbal Tea
- 1/2 cup of raspberries
- 1/2 cup blueberries
- 1/2 burro banana
- One tablespoon of date sugar or agave syrup

Instructions:

1. To prepare your "brain-boosting" smoothie, start by boiling one cup of distilled water and add 1/2 tablespoon of Dr. Sebi's Nerve / Stress Relief Herbal Tea. Steep for 10 - 15 minutes, strain. Let cool.
2. Once the tea is cooled, blend in a high-speed blender along with the rest of the ingredients.
3. Enjoy!

DINNER - ONE-POT ZUCCHINI MUSHROOM PASTA

Ingredients:

- 1 pound approved-grain spaghetti (like spelled or Kamut)
- 1 pound cremini mushrooms, thinly sliced
- Two zucchini, thinly sliced and quartered
- Two sprigs thyme
- Sea salt and cayenne pepper, to taste
- 1/4 cup homemade walnut milk

Instructions:

1. In a large stockpot or Dutch oven, over medium-high heat, combine spaghetti, mushrooms, zucchini, and thyme and 4 1/2 cups water; season with sea salt cayenne pepper, to taste.
2. Bring to a boil; reduce heat and simmer, uncovered, until pasta is cooked through and liquid has reduced about 8-10 minutes.
3. Stir in homemade walnut milk.
4. Serve immediately and enjoy it.

DAY 21

BREAKFAST - DR. SEBI'S SEA MOSS PANNA COTTA

Ingredients:

- 2/3 cup soaked walnuts
- 2 cups + 2 tablespoons soft-jelly coconut water
- One tablespoon of Bromide Plus Powder
- ½ heaping cup soft-jelly young coconut meat
- ¼ cup agave syrup
- Pinch unrefined sea salt
- ¼ cup + 1 tablespoon coconut oil

Instructions:

1. To prepare your sea moss panna cotta, begin by blending (preferably in a high-speed blender) the soaked walnuts and soft-jelly coconut water.
2. Blend at medium-high speed until very smooth. Strain through a nut milk bag or line a strainer with a double layer of cheesecloth and pour through. Squeeze to remove as much liquid as possible.
3. In a high-speed blender, place the walnut milk you just made, Bromide Plus Powder, soft-jelly coconut meat, and agave syrup.
4. Blend at medium speed, and then increase to high speed until completely smooth. These would take 1 to 2 minutes. Make sure the mixture is completely smooth.
5. Grease the insides of 6 ramekins, molds, or espresso cups with coconut oil (if you plan to serve in the ramekins/cups, no need to grease). Pour mixture in to fill to the desired height. Chill your sea moss panna cotta in the fridge for at least 2 hours or until set and firm.
6. Add strawberries and agave syrup to taste before serving. Enjoy!

LUNCH - DR. SEBI'S HEAVY METAL DETOX SMOOTHIE

Ingredients:

- One burro banana
- 1-2 cups blueberries
- 1 cup Seville orange juice
- 1 cup watercress
- One organic apple
- One tablespoon of Dr. Sebi's Bromide Plus Powder
- 1 cup spring water

Instructions:

1. To prepare the heavy metal detox smoothie, blend all ingredients in a high-speed blender until smooth.
2. If a thinner consistency is desired, add up to 1 cup of water. Enjoy!

DINNER - DR. SEBI'S "OWL" BLUEBERRY PANCAKES

Ingredients:

- 1 1/4 cup homemade walnut milk
- 1 1/2 cup spelled, amaranth, or Kamut flour
- 3 tbsp. date sugar
- One pinch sea salt
- 2 tbsp. grapeseed oil
- 1/3 cup blueberries
- Agave syrup and extra fruit for serving

Instructions:

1. To prepare Dr. Sebi's plant-based "owl" blueberry pancakes, begin by whisking together flour and date sugar to eliminate any lumps. Pour homemade walnut milk and grape seed oil into the flour/date sugar mixture and whisk until lumpy but with flour mostly integrated.
2. Add blueberries and fold in with a spatula to maintain lumps. DO NOT OVERMIX.
3. Preheat griddle to 350F (or a large pan to medium heat) and brush on an even, a light coating of grapeseed oil.
4. Add 1/4-1/3 cup servings of the pancake batter to the griddle. Gently flatten with a spoon/ladle back to the desired shape and even out the batter.
5. Cook for about 2-3 minutes until the edges are slightly cooked and the bottom is golden.
6. Flip and cook for another minute or two until that side is golden as well.
7. Serve with agave syrup and extra fruit to make the "owl" shapes.

DAY 22

BREAKFAST - DR. SEBI'S FANTASTIC QUINOA BREAD

Ingredients:

- 300 g (10 ½ oz or 1 3/4 cups) whole uncooked quinoa seed
- 1/2 cup water
- 60 ml (2 fl oz / ¼ cup) grapeseed oil
- 1/2 teaspoon sea salt
- 1/2 key lime, juiced

Instructions:

1. Soak quinoa in plenty of cold water overnight in the fridge. Preheat oven to 160 C / 320 F.
2. Drain the quinoa and rinse well through a sieve. Make sure the water is fully drained from your sieve. Place the quinoa into a food processor.
3. Add ½ cup of water, grape seed oil, sea salt, and key lime juice.
4. Mix in a food processor for 3 minutes. The bread mix should resemble a batter consistency with some whole quinoa still left in the mix.
5. Spoon into a loaf tin lined with baking paper on all sides and the base.
6. Bake for 1 ½ hour until firm to touch and bounces back when pressed with your fingers.
7. Remove from the oven and cool for 30 minutes in the tin, then remove from the tin and cool completely on a rack. The bread should be slightly moist in the middle and crisp on the outside.
8. Cool completely before eating and enjoy

LUNCH - ALL-NATURAL TAMARIND PASTE

Ingredients:

- 250 gr of natural tamarind
- 3 cups of spring water

Instructions:

1. Clean the tamarind. Check for any seeds, skin, or unwanted particles and discard them. Meanwhile, heat 2 cups of water.
2. Soak the tamarind in 2 cups of hot water for about 45-60 minutes.
3. Once the tamarind is soft, blend in a high-speed blender until very smooth.
4. Pass the resulting mixture through a sifter. Discard any stones, seeds, or debris.

5. Boil the resulting pulp for 5 minutes over medium flame.

6. Once the pasta is completely cooled, store in airtight containers.

DINNER - DR. SEBI'S CREAMY VEGETABLE SOUP

Ingredients:

- One tablespoon grapeseed oil
- 1/4 of a yellow onion
- One bell pepper (red)
- One zucchini
- Cayenne pepper, to taste
- Sea salt, to taste
- Approved herbs (optional)
- 1 cup homemade walnut milk

Instructions:

1. In a large pot, sauté the chopped onion in the grapeseed oil until the onion is translucent.

2. Add the chopped pepper and zucchini and cook over medium heat for about 5 minutes.

3. When the vegetables are soft, blend with the homemade walnut milk.

4. Simmer for 15 minutes. Season to taste.

5. Serve with fresh approved herbs.

DAY 23

BREAKFAST - HEALTHY "FRIED-RICE"

Ingredients:

- 1 cup cooked wild rice or quinoa
- 1/2 cup sliced bell peppers
- 1/2 cup sliced mushrooms
- 1/2 cup sliced zucchini
- 1/4 onion, cubed
- 1 tbsp. grapeseed oil
- Sea salt and cayenne pepper, to taste

Instructions:

1. Heat oil in a pan, and sautée onion until browned.
2. Add remaining vegetables and cook for another 5 minutes. Make sure they're not too soft.
3. Add the cup of boiled rice, and continue cooking until lightly browned.

LUNCH - VEGGIE FAJITAS TACOS

Time Taken: 15 minutes!

Ingredients:

- 2-3 large portobello mushrooms
- Two bell peppers
- One onion
- Juice of 1/2 key lime
- 1 Tbsp. grapeseed oil
- Six corn-free tortillas (look for tortillas made with approved grains, like these Kamut flour tortillas)
- Your choice of approved seasonings (onion powder, habanero, cayenne pepper)
- Avocado

Instructions:

1. Remove stems of mushrooms, spoon out gills if desired, and wipe tops clean. Cut into about 1/3 inch thick slices.
2. Thinly slice bell peppers and onion.
3. In a large skillet over medium heat, add 1 Tbsp. Grape seed oil and peppers and onions. Cook for about 2 minutes.
4. Add mushrooms and seasonings. Stir occasionally, cook another 7-8 minutes or until softened.
5. Warm tortillas and spoon the fajita mixture into the center of tortillas. Serve with avocado and key lime juice.

DINNER - CLASSIC HOMEMADE HUMMUS

Ingredients:

- 1 cup cooked chickpeas
- 1/3 cup homemade tahini butter
- 2 tbsp. olive oil
- 2 tbsp. key lime juice
- A dash of onion powder
- Sea salt, to taste

Instructions:

- Blend all the ingredients in a food processor or high-powered blender, and serve.

DAY 24

BREAKFAST - JUICY PORTOBELLO BURGERS

Ingredients:

- Two large portobello mushroom caps
- 3 tbsp. olive oil
- 2 tsp. dried basil
- 1 tsp. dried oregano
- 1/2 tsp. Cayenne pepper
- One tomato sliced
- One avocado sliced
- 1 cup purslane

Instructions:

1. Slice the mushroom stems off and slice off about 1/2" of the mushroom top (as if slicing a bun).
2. Combine olive oil, onion powder, basil, oregano, and Cayenne pepper in a small bowl and mix well.
3. Place mushroom caps on a cookie sheet with foil and a little grapeseed oil (to prevent sticking).
4. With a large spoon, pour marinade over each mushroom cap and allow to sit about 10 mins.
5. Preheat oven to 425*F and bake mushrooms for about 10 mins; check the preparedness level before flipping them to bake another 10 mins.
6. Place the bottom of the mushroom cap on a plate - add your choice of toppings - and top with the top portion of the baked mushroom cap.

LUNCH - THE GRILLED ROMAINE LETTUCE SALAD

Ingredients:

- Four small heads of romaine lettuce, rinsed
- 1 tbsp. red onion, chopped finely
- 1 tbsp. key lime juice
- Onion powder, to taste
- 1 tbsp. fresh basil, chopped
- Sea salt and cayenne pepper, to taste
- 4 tbsp. olive oil
- 1 tbsp. agave syrup

Instructions:

1. Place lettuce halves cut side down in a large nonstick pan. Don't add any oil. Check the color of the lettuce by turning them. Make sure the lettuce is browned on both sides.
2. Take the pan off the heat and allow lettuce to cool on a large platter.
3. For the dressing, combine red onion with olive oil, agave syrup, key lime juice, and fresh basil in a small mixing bowl. Add salt and cayenne pepper to taste. Whisk well to combine.
4. Transfer grilled lettuce onto a serving dish and drizzle with the dressing.
5. Enjoy!

Instructions:

1. Soak wakame stems for 5-10 minutes and drain.
2. In a mixing bowl, combine sesame oil, agave syrup, key lime juice, onion powder, and ginger. Whisk thoroughly.
3. Place wakame and bell pepper in a serving dish. Pour dressing on top.
4. Sprinkle with sesame seeds and enjoy!

DINNER - WAKAME SALAD

Ingredients:

- 2 cups wakame stems (you can use other sea vegetables, as long as they appear on Dr. Sebi's Nutritional Guide)
- 1 tsp. onion powder
- 1 tsp. ginger
- 1 tbsp. red bell pepper
- 1 tbsp. sesame seeds
- 1 tbsp. key lime juice
- 1 tbsp. agave syrup
- 1 tbsp. sesame oil

DAY 25

BREAKFAST - BERRY SORBET

Ingredients:

- 1/2 cup date sugar
- 1 1/2 tsp. spelled flour
- 2 cups strawberries (pureed)
- 2 cups of water

Instructions:

1. Dissolve the date sugar and flour in the water in a large saucepan over low heat, then boil until thick, like syrup, about ten minutes. Remove from the heat and cool.
2. When the syrup is completely cooled, add the pureed fruit and mix well.
3. Cut the sorbet into chunks, then process in a blender or food processor until smooth and creamy.
4. Place in a plastic container and freeze uncovered until it is solid.
5. Put the sorbet back into the freezer and allow to freeze for another 4 hours.

LUNCH - CHAMOMILE DELIGHT SMOOTHIE

Ingredients:

- One burro banana
- 1/4 cup prepared Dr. Sebi's Nerve/Stress Relief Herbal Tea
- 1/2 cup homemade walnut milk
- 1 tbsp. date sugar

Instructions:

1. Wait for the tea to cool.
2. Blend with the rest of the ingredients and enjoy!

DINNER - DR. SEBI'S ENERGIZER SMOOTHIE

Ingredients:

- 1 cup cubed papaya or melon
- 1 cup homemade hemp milk
- 1/2 cup cooked quinoa or amaranth
- One date or 1 tbsp. date sugar
- 1 tsp. Bromide Plus Powder

Instructions:

- Blend all the ingredients and enjoy!

DAY 26

BREAKFAST - DR. SEBI'S ORANGE CREAMSICLE SMOOTHIE

Ingredients:

- 3 Seville oranges, peeled
- 1/2 Burro banana
- 1 cup of coconut water
- Date sugar, to taste
- 1/2 tsp. Bromide Plus Powder

Instructions:

- Add all the ingredients to your blender and blend until smooth. Serve and enjoy

LUNCH - STEWED OKRA AND TOMATOES

Ingredients:

- 2 cups fresh okra
- 1 cup cherry tomatoes
- One medium onion
- One tablespoon avocado oil
- 1/2 cup fresh spring water
- Sea salt and cayenne pepper, to taste

Instructions:

1. Peel and dice the onion and cherry tomatoes.
2. Heat the avocado oil in a skillet, and add the chopped onion. Cook until the onion becomes translucent.
3. Once the onions become translucent, add the okra and spring water. Cook for 10 minutes over low heat.
4. Add the chopped cherry tomatoes and simmer for an additional 20 minutes or until okra is cooked through.
5. Add sea salt and pepper to taste.

DINNER - DR. SEBI'S CHICKPEA LOAF

Ingredients:

- 1 1/2 cups of finely diced onions
- Two bell peppers, finely diced
- Two tablespoons grapeseed oil
- 1/2 cup minced fresh basil

- Two tablespoons + 1/2 teaspoon homemade natural granulated onion
- One teaspoon sea salt
- 3/4 teaspoon dried sage
- 1/2 teaspoon dried oregano
- 1/2 teaspoon cayenne pepper
- 1/4 teaspoon dried thyme
- 3 cups chickpeas, cooked
- 1 cup mushrooms (all kinds, except shiitake)
- 1/2 cup spelled flour
- Sea salt and cayenne pepper, to taste

Instructions:

1. Preheat oven to 350 °F.
2. In a large pan, sauté mushrooms, bell peppers, and onion in grapeseed oil over medium-high heat for 2 to 3 minutes.
3. Stir in minced basil and remove from heat. Stir in seasonings.
4. Coarsely chop chickpeas in a food processor or by hand. Stir into sautéed vegetables. Add spelled flour and mix well.
5. Grease a loaf pan with grapeseed oil. Bake uncovered at 350 °F for 55 to 60 minutes.

DAY 27

BREAKFAST - MAGNESIUM-BOOSTING SMOOTHIE

Ingredients:

- 1 cup fresh spring water
- 1/4 cup Brazil Nuts
- 1/2 burro banana
- Two strawberries
- 1/2 cup figs

Instructions:

1. Blend all ingredients in a high-speed blender.
2. Add more water if the mixture is too thick
3. Enjoy!

LUNCH - ALKALINE-ELECTRIC CLASSIC APPLE BAKE

Ingredients:

- 3 - 4 Gala or Honey crisp apples, depending on how big they are. (read about our choice of apples here)
- Three tablespoons agave syrup
- One tablespoon chopped walnuts
- Pinch of cloves

Instructions:

1. To prepare this classic apple bake, start by preheating the oven to 350 degrees. Slice apples thinly. Place in a large bowl and drizzle with agave syrup. Stir well to coat evenly.
2. Combine cloves and walnuts and sprinkle over agave coated apples, stirring while sprinkling to coat. Let set about 5 minutes to encourage the juices to come out.
3. Arrange sliced apples into a casserole dish.
4. Bake for 15 minutes, then cover with foil and bake another 35-40 minutes, or until apples are bubbly and your kitchen smells amazing!

DINNER - PLANT-BASED QUINOA BOWL

Ingredients:

- 1 cup cooked quinoa

- One handful of approved greens
- One tablespoon of grapeseed oil
- Two cups chopped approved vegetables, such as zucchini, cherry tomatoes, bell pepper, etc.
- Sea salt and cayenne pepper, to taste

Instructions:

1. In a large pan, heat a tablespoon of grapeseed oil. Sautee the chopped vegetables until tender.
2. Mix the vegetables with the cooked quinoa and the fresh greens.
3. Season with sea salt and cayenne pepper to taste.

DAY 28

BREAKFAST - GREEN PANCAKES

Ingredients:

- 1/2 cup chickpea flour
- 1/2 teaspoon sea salt
- 1/2 cup fresh spring water
- 1/4 cup blueberries
- One burro banana
- One tablespoon agave syrup
- One handful of amaranth greens
- One tablespoon of your preferred nut butter for extra protein (homemade tahini, or homemade walnut or Brazil nut butter)

Instructions:

1. Add all of the ingredients to a blender and mix until smooth. Be careful not to add too much water, or they won't be as fluffy or cook as well.
2. Let the batter sit for 5-10 minutes. While it's resting, heat a nonstick frying pan over medium-high heat.
3. Scoop the batter into the pan to form 6 small pancakes. You can vary the size if you want. It should make either three large pancakes, 4-5 medium ones, or six small ones.
4. Let them cook until there are some bubbles in the batter, and they're starting to look fluffy and cooked around the edges. Flip and cook for another couple of minutes.
5. Serve decorated with blueberries, burro banana, and agave syrup. Enjoy your Green Pancakes!

LUNCH - DR. SEBI'S NO-BAKE ENERGY BALLS

Ingredients:

- 3/4 cup raspberries
- Ten dates
- 1 cup walnuts
- 2 2/3 cup shredded soft-jelly coconut meat
- One pinch of sea salt

Instructions:

1. To make Dr. Sebi's No-Bake Energy Balls, put all ingredients in a food processor or blender. Process or blend until all ingredients are combined.
2. Use moist hands to form the no-bake energy balls.
3. When all balls have been formed, place the tray in the freezer for 20-30 minutes.
4. Enjoy!

DINNER - DR. SEBI'S MANGO SALAD

Ingredients:

- Two mangoes
- 1/4 red onion
- 1/4 cup cherry tomatoes
- 1/2 cucumber, seeded
- 1/2 green bell pepper
- One key lime
- Sea salt and cayenne pepper, to taste.

Instructions:

1. To prepare your Mango Salad, start by cutting the mangoes, cherry tomatoes, and red onion into small cubes.
2. Slice the seeded cucumber and the bell pepper finely.
3. Mix all ingredients in a small bowl. Juice the key lime and pour over the salad.
4. Season with sea salt and pepper and let marinate in the fridge for at least 20 minutes before eating.
5. Enjoy as a salad, salsa, or dip, and it's your call!

DAY 29

BREAKFAST - PLANT-BASED CHICKPEA QUINOA BURGERS

Ingredients:

- 1/4 chopped onion
- 1 1/2 cup cooked chickpeas (garbanzo beans)
- 1 1/2 cups cooked quinoa
- 1/4 cup cooked amaranth
- Two tablespoons fresh (approved) herbs of your choice
- Two tablespoons water
- Sea salt and cayenne pepper, to taste
- Vegetables of your choice for serving: cherry tomatoes, green (approved) leaves like wild arugula, watercress or lettuce, etc.
- One tablespoon per patty of raw homemade sesame "tahini" butter

Instructions:

1. Preheat the oven to 375 degrees F.
2. Place the onion and herbs in a food processor. Pulse until they are finely chopped. Add your chickpeas, quinoa, and amaranth, and continue to pulse. Don't puree the mixture; you want it to be a little chunky.
3. Add sea salt and cayenne pepper, and process until a dough begins to form. Add water while the food processor is running, and the dough comes together. You want the mixture to be sticky, not runny or dry. Place the bowl in the refrigerator and let cool for 15 minutes.
4. Once chilled, separate the mixture into eight equal-sized patties.
5. Place your patties on a parchment paper-lined baking sheet and bake for 20 minutes. Flip halfway through and finish with a quick 2 - 3-minute broil to get the patties nice and browned.
6. Serve in an approved-flour bun with homemade raw sesame "tahini" butter and wild arugula, watercress, or lettuce.

LUNCH - ALKALINE-ELECTRIC ICE CREAM

Ingredients:

- Two ripe mangoes
- Two burro bananas
- Three tablespoons of homemade walnut milk
- Agave syrup or date sugar (optional).

Instructions:

1. Peel and cut the mangoes into cubes. Peel the burro bananas as well, and slice.
2. Put the mango and banana pieces in a baking sheet lined with parchment paper. Freeze.
3. Place your frozen fruit into the bowl of a food processor or powerful blender. Add the homemade walnut milk and the sweetener (optional).
4. Blend for approx. 3 - 4 minutes. It will look like it's never going to go ice-creamy but stick with it. You might need to stop it throughout to push it down the sides and stir it around a bit.

Instructions:

1. In a pan, pour a tablespoon of grapeseed oil and sauteé onions and peppers until they are tender.
2. In a large bowl, mix the sauteed vegetables with the rest of the ingredients.
3. Form patties with your hands, cook them in a skillet for about 3 minutes on each side, or crispy.
4. Enjoy!

DINNER - TEF GRAIN BURGERS

Ingredients

- 1 1/2 cups cooked tef grain
- 1 1/2 cups garbanzo bean (chickpea) flour
- 1/4 of an onion, diced
- 1/4 cup bell peppers, finely diced
- One teaspoon oregano
- One teaspoon basil
- One teaspoon dill
- One tablespoon grapeseed oil
- Sea salt and cayenne pepper, to taste

DAY 30

BREAKFAST - ALKALINE-ELECTRIC SPRING SALAD

Ingredients:

- 4 cups seasonal approved greens of your choice (wild arugula, dandelion greens, watercress)
- 1 cup cherry tomatoes
- 1/4 cup walnuts
- 1/4 cup approved herbs of your choice (dill, sweet basil, etc.)

For the dressing:

- 3-4 key limes
- One tablespoon of homemade raw sesame "tahini" butter
- Sea salt and cayenne pepper, to taste

Instructions:

1. Juice the key limes.
2. In a small bowl, whisk together the key lime juice with the homemade raw sesame "tahini" butter. Add sea salt and cayenne pepper, to taste.
3. Cut the cherry tomatoes in half.
4. In a large bowl, combine the greens, cherry tomatoes, and herbs. Pour the dressing on top and "massage" with your hands.
5. Let the greens soak up the dressing. Add more sea salt, cayenne pepper, and herbs on top if you wish. Enjoy

LUNCH - IMMUNITY-BOOSTING SMOOTHIE

Ingredients:

- 1/2 mango
- 1 Seville orange
- 1 cup brewed Dr. Sebi's Immune Support Herbal Tea
- One tablespoon coconut oil
- One tablespoon date sugar or agave syrup
- One key lime, juiced

Instructions:

1. Boil two cups of distilled water and add 1 ½ tablespoon of Dr. Sebi's Immune Support Herbal Tea. Simmer for about 15 minutes. Allow to cool, strain.
2. Peel the Seville orange and cut the mango into chunks.

3. Blend all the ingredients in a high-speed blender. Enjoy!

DINNER - PLANT-BASED MUSHROOM GRAVY!

Ingredients:

- Two tablespoons grapeseed oil
- 1/4 of an onion, diced
- 1 cup thinly sliced mushrooms (any type, except shiitake)
- One pinch each sea salt and cayenne pepper
- 1 1/2 tablespoons amaranth or spelled flour
- 1/2 cup homemade (approved) vegetable broth
- 1 cup homemade walnut milk
- Two tablespoons of finely chopped walnuts
- 1/2 teaspoon fresh thyme

Instructions:

1. Add grapeseed oil to a cast-iron skillet or large saucepan over medium heat. Then onion and mushrooms and season with a pinch each sea salt and cayenne pepper. Cook for 3-4 minutes or until the onions are translucent.
2. Add amaranth or spelled flour and whisk to coat. Cook for 1 minute.
3. Then slowly whisk in homemade vegetable broth and walnut milk, starting with 1/2 cup walnut milk and building up. Season again with a pinch each sea salt and cayenne pepper. Cook until thickened, frequently stirring, over low heat. Taste and adjust seasonings as needed.
4. Add walnuts and stir to combine. Keep on low until you're ready to serve, adding more walnut milk as needed if it gets too thick.
5. Serve over plant-based biscuits or bread made with flour from approved grains.

DR SEBI'S CELL FOOD SUPPLEMENT

THE WHOLE FOOD SUPPLEMENT

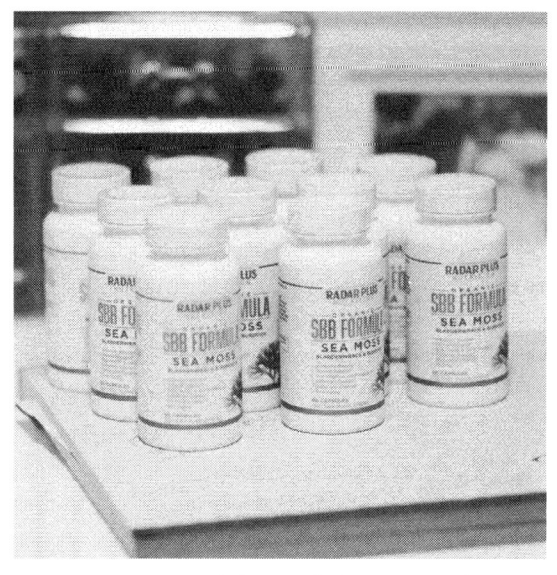

The effect of whole food supplements has been very favorably contrasted with artificial supplements such as multivitamins. The reason whole food supplements come out on top is simple: our body recognizes the ratios of nutrients in whole foods. It processes them far more easily than supplements consisting of isolated or fractionated nutrients. The body recognizes whole food supplements as nutritional and can metabolize and utilize them efficiently.

The best idea, say, experts, when it comes to determining your whole food supplements requirements is to decide on the readily available foods you can and will eat consistently and fill in the gaps. A general list of the most highly recommended vegetables regarding anti-aging and health benefits would include Kale, chard, spinach, broccoli, Brussels sprouts, cauliflower, red and green peppers, garlic, onions, sweet potatoes, tomatoes, green peas, asparagus, and carrots.

WHAT SUPPLEMENTS SHOULD YOU TAKE?

Whether you use vital nutrients as your barometer of what and how much to eat or as a guide in determining what whole food supplements you need, determining their presence or lack thereof is probably the best way to evaluate a diet. Below are some of the vital supplements most should consider alongside their diet, as recommended by Dr. Sebi.

> **Banju**: Dr. Sebi's Banju provides targeted nutrition and cleansing for the brain and nervous system. The tonic is rich in potassium phosphate to replenish minerals and antioxidants, reducing neurological inflammation.
> - Elderberry delivers a spectrum of flavonoids that protect and nourish the brain, enhancing neurological energy metabolism.

- Blue Vervain delivers emotional and nervous restoration, reducing anxiety and relieving tension.
- Burdock Root purifies and unifies the blood, increasing iron and oxygenation.
- Valerian Root calms the nervous system: aiding peaceful and restful sleep, reducing irritability, and soothing pain.
- The astringent Bugleweed supports detoxification and nourishes endocrine glands governing energy metabolism.

The tonic enhances focus and cognitive functions, stabilizes emotions, balances the nervous system, and protects against oxidative stress.

Viento: Dr. Sebi's Viento is energizing, cleansing, and revitalizing.
- Enhancing circulation and oxygenation, the iron-rich capsules increase mental energy and physical stamina.
- Chaparral supports lymphatic waste removal and expulsion of energy-draining heavy metals.
- The potent antioxidant lignans reduce inflammatory damage, enhance immune defenses, and reduce addictive cravings.
- Bladderwrack's nutritive iodides and cleansing bromides boost thyroid function, improving oxygen levels, energy regulation, and reducing appetite.
- Valerian and Toad's Herb improve circulation, reduce stress, increase cellular oxygenation, and free up energy for vital immune functions.
- Quassia Amara encourages the creation of oxygen-carrying red blood cells, enhancing cellular nutrition and energy production.
- Invigorating herbs support your body's natural energy efficiency, boosting emotional stability, and mental clarity.

Testo: Dr. Sebi's Testo boosts testosterone and enhances sexual virility. The potent herbs have helped thousands of men enhance sexual stamina, increase erectile strength, and reclaim sexual drive and desire.

- Sarsaparilla vine, an aphrodisiac native to Honduras, increases blood flow, helping the penis get engorged.
- Yohimbe, a West African sexual enhancer, contains testosterone-boosting alkaloids, enhancing vigor.
- Locust Bark's antioxidants and glycosides reduce inflammation and improve erectile blood flow.
- Capadulla, a Caribbean aphrodisiac, nourishes the whole urogenital system, preventing sexual decline.
- Irish Sea Moss is a remineralizing aphrodisiac, used since Roman times.
- Nopal supports the prostate, reducing inflammation and enhancing testosterone levels.
- Muira Puama stimulates libido and improves genital blood flow, naturally increasing penis sensation.

Iron Plus: Dr. Sebi's Iron Plus is a nourishing and cleansing tonic that supports the blood and immune system. Antioxidants mitigate inflammation and help the immune system focus on rejuvenation.

- Elderberry's indigo-blue pigments mitigate free radical damage and reduce mucus.
- Blue Vervain & Chaparral, used traditionally by Native Americans, support digestive and respiratory functions.
- Hombre Grande and Quassia help purge parasites, mucus, and putrid waste from the bowel, while Palo Guaco reduces intestinal inflammation.
- Bugleweed's astringent aromatic bitters encourage detoxification and reduce endocrine inflammation.
- Cardo Santo, known as blessed thistle, regulates appetite, soothes indigestion, and helps regulate blood pressure.

Bio Ferro Tonic: Dr. Sebi's Bio Ferro Tonic nourishes and cleanses the blood, supporting your immune system. Saturated with minerals and bioactive plant compounds, this liquid formulation provides deep cellular nutrition.

- Elderberry's rich indigo-blue flavonoids reduce inflammation.
- Chaparral used traditionally for arthritis helps remove toxins from the blood.
- Burdock's deep roots cleanse the blood, delivering oxygenating iron.
- Yellow Dock supports the circulatory system, reducing inflammation and blood pressure.
- Anti-inflammatory Cocolmeca promotes waste excretion and protects against cholesterol oxidation.
- Muicle helps cells respond to insulin, aiding blood sugar balance.
- Blue Vervain promotes restorative immune functions and reduces stress.
- Encino contains antioxidants targeting blood vessel inflammation.

Estro: Dr. Sebi's Estro supports female reproductive health and hormonal balance. Targeted antioxidants and aphrodisiacs support libido and ease menstruation.

- Hydrangea's flavonoids, saponins, and essential oils nourish the urogenital system while renowned aphrodisiac, Damiana, increases genital blood flow and sensitivity.
- Anti-inflammatory Sarsaparilla reduces pain and enhances detoxification.
- Irish Sea Moss balances the thyroid gland, while Muscle supports the production of new blood.
- Red Clover reduces hot flashes, soothes breast tenderness, and eases premenstrual or menopausal symptoms while relaxing.
- Blue Vervain reduces cramps.
- Muira Puama stimulates sexual desire and increases stamina.
- Abuta purifies the blood and stabilizes hormones, promoting emotional balance.

The potent herbs increase female sexual satisfaction, vaginal lubrication, and hormonal balance.

PART THREE

MAINTENANCE PROGRAM: FOOD PLAN FOR WEIGHT MAINTENANCE

HOW TO DEVELOP SUCCESSFUL STRATEGIES FOR WEIGHT MAINTENANCE AFTER WEIGHT LOSS?

Losing weight on a low carbohydrate diet can be relatively easy, but what happens when we finish the diet? You are now left trying to maintain the bodyweight you are comfortable with. It is so easy to go back to old habits, and ways of eating that will result in you putting the pounds back on. I believe it is those people that make an effort to develop strategies to organize and plan their daily diet who are going to be those who will have the most success at maintaining their weight.

The single most effective strategy to develop is your mindset, making or breaking your continuing maintenance diet after losing weight. Ultimately your success will depend on what is going on in your mind. Weight gain is often more about what goes on in your mind than what goes into your mouth.

A good mindset is important, but you need to make sure that you are fully informed. This can be achieved by understanding what good food choices are; the best way to achieve this by researching the subject. For example, reading every book can get hold of on the library's low carbohydrate diet lifestyle. Surfing the net, by typing into the search engine the words, low carbohydrate diets, then visiting the blogs and websites that come up in the search.

Measure your performance. This can be done by weighing yourself regularly. I like to weigh myself every day, but you may prefer to weigh weekly. There are other ways of tracking your performance; for example, if you don't want to weigh yourself, you could instead see how comfortably you fit into a pair of trousers or skirt that is your maintenance target size. Another alternative to weighing yourself is to measure your waist using a tape measure frequently. The method you use to monitor your weight does not matter, and the important thing is to measure your performance regularly.

Use charts, trackers, and meal planners to record your performance and goals, which will help keep you motivated and on target. When I weigh myself daily, I quickly jot the weight down on a calendar I have hanging on the wall.

That's why I decided to give you a great and useful gift!

At the end of this book, you'll find included:

"**Dr. Sebi Journal: 30 Days to Detox and Improve Yourself. In this motivation journal based on Dr. Sebi's plant-based alkaline diet, you can keep track of your meals, goals, and progress**" by *Elizabeth Bowman*, a 30-day based journal where you can write down all of your steps to wellness and detoxification.

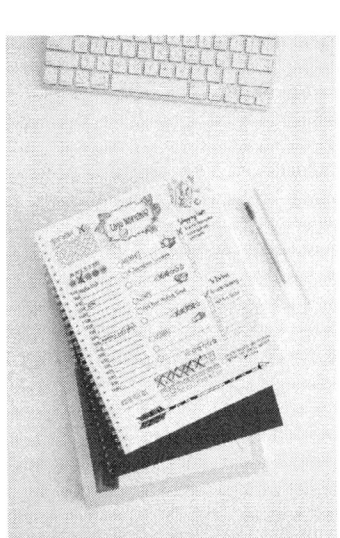
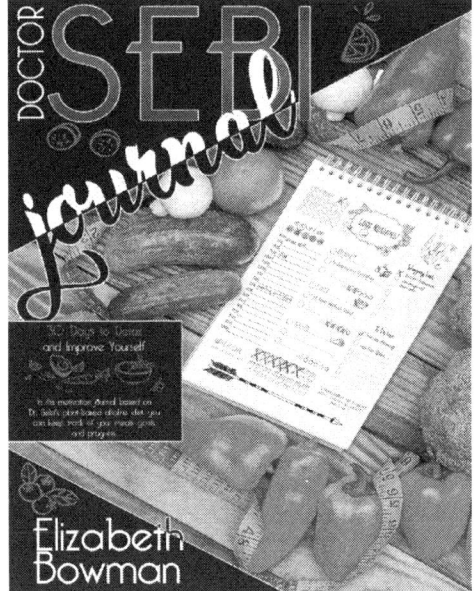
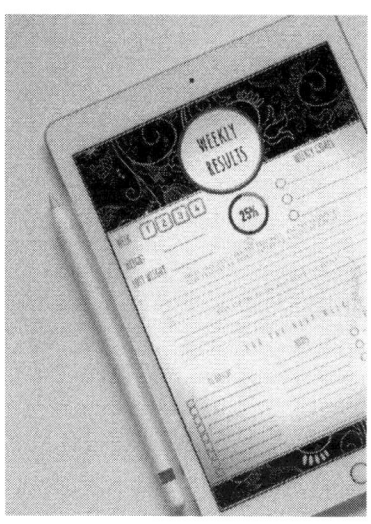

You'll be able to write down all of your daily meals, shopping list, thoughts, goals, and successes.

You will find inside all the instructions to do so.

You'll be able to fill out your daily plan directly in the book or download a printable version at the link you see below to use the planner all year round as well.

https://BookHip.com/LGQXHHH

Develop and cultivate new healthy eating habits. These can include eating regular meals and fewer snacks and preparing most meals at home rather than eating in restaurants or eating from fast food outlets. Try monitoring your intake by counting carbs.

Think of strategies you could use to tackle stress and other emotional problems in ways that do not involve food or drink. It may be that you have turned to food throughout your life to help you cope through difficult or stressful times. For example, you could try expressing your feelings by talking to somebody, instead of internalizing your emotions and turning to food.

Find ways of increasing the amount of exercise you get during the day. These could be as simple as walking upstairs instead of taking the elevator, taking the dogs out for walks, taking the kids to the park, walk instead of taking the car for short trips. You may also want to consider organized exercise. Perhaps joining a gym or taking up yoga, exercise classes, or dance classes.

I hope that by following some of my suggestions, you will be successful in maintaining your weight. Following a low carbohydrate maintenance diet and follow the food recommended by Dr. Sebi, can be an excellent way to maintain your body at the weight you want.

I wish you every success.

CONCLUSIONS

We as an individual realize that eating out can be challenging when trying to follow an entire food, plant-based diet and maintaining a strategic distance from oil and other concentrated fixings or on the off chance that you have to eat without gluten as recommended by Dr. Sebi. Then again, requesting takeout or dine-in can be quite convenient after a long, stressed, and hectic day where processed food was basically not in your arrangements. In this way, here are a few tips you can utilize when eating out.

- Look into specialty restaurants, for example, plant-based eateries or vegetarian restaurants.
- Determine how you need your dinners arranged. Always opt for steamed, heated, water sautéed or barbecued
- Get along with the stand by staff to get them to cause your inclinations to occur.

It's clear now to see how a plant-based diet's way of life can be advantageous for your health rather than proceed with a vegan diet. I trust that the book addressed all inquiries you may have caught wind of this way of slimming down and that you can begin to make it work for you. If you are as yet reluctant about completely surrendering animal products, you don't need to. The fundamental remove here is that you make plant-based supreme principle part of your diet as you make gradual steps to progress into a full plant-based way of life. You will soon understand that your body and mind begin to feel good, stronger, healthier, and more advantageous.

You can't fix your well-being until you fix your diet!

ABOUT THE AUTHOR

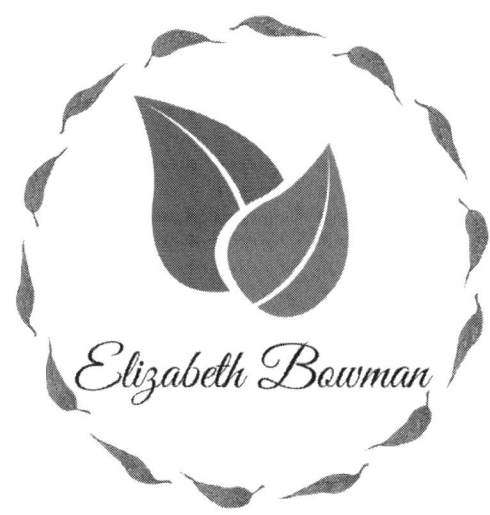

BIOGRAPHY

Elizabeth Bowman is an American author born and raised in the great state of Texas. While stumbling around in search of her true course in life she began to notice the state of those around her.

Everywhere she went Elizabeth noticed masses of people with obviously unhealthy lifestyles. She went back to college and earned a Bachelors in Dietetics from Baylor University.

Elizabeth spent several years working in different practices before opening her own business. Her one passion in life is from helping others achieve their weight-loss goals while retraining their minds to enjoy a cleaner, healthy existence.

Elizabeth specializes in alternative diets with an emphasis on vegan. She has tailored her programs to include the total package, with focuses on losing weight and keeping it off, and a combination of mental health and physical wellbeing.

Her bestselling book, Dr. Sebi Diet: Plant Based Meal Plan for Sustainable Weight Loss. Detox Your Body with Healthy Lifestyle Based Diets and Boost Your Energy Through the Day is available everywhere.

Her belief that having knowledge is only as important as sharing it is conveyed in all she does. Elizabeth is generous and caring, showing genuine concern for her patients as she helps them traverse the often difficult course back to better health.

She has helped thousands of patients over the course of her career and plans to continue until Father Time gets the better of her.

Elizabeth is the proud mother of two adult women and a devoted wife of over thirty years. To relax and unwind she enjoy long walks with her husband and their dogs, yoga, meditation, and reading. The inspiration for clean living prompted her to seek out innovative and unique recipes for the whole family.

BOOKS BY ELIZABETH BOWMAN

- 2020
  - *Dr. Sebi Diet: Plant-Based Meal Plan for Sustainable Weight-Loss. Detox Your Body with Healthy Lifestyle Based Diets and Boost Your Energy Through the Day*
- 2021
  - *Dr. Sebi Diet: The complete guide to the Sebi Plant-Based Diet. How to eliminate mucus from your body, detox and prevent disease with alkaline food list. 2021 Edition with 30-Day Printable Journal!*
  - *Dr. Sebi Detox: The step by step 30-Day Meal Plan to cleanse and lose weight based on Doctor Sebi's alkaline plant-based diet. Weight maintenance program and 30-Day Printable Journal included!*
  - *Dr.Sebi Journal: 30 Days to Detox and Improve Yourself. In this motivation journal based on Dr. Sebi's plant-based alkaline diet, you can keep track of your meals, goals, and progress.*

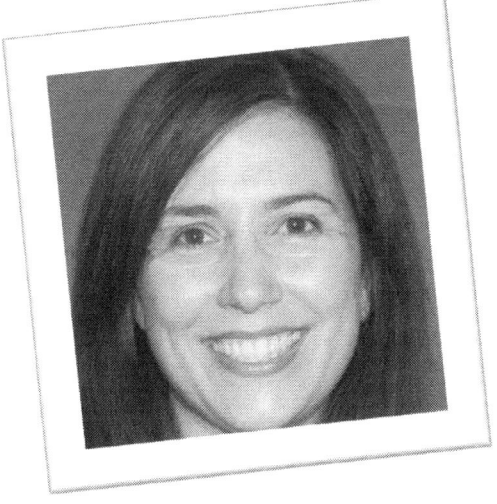

"…Hi I'm Elizabeth!

I live through the publication of my books, if you liked this guide, I invite you to write an **honest review** and visit my author page.

Thank you"

Elizabeth Bowman

Want more? Grab *Dr. Sebi Journal: 30 Days to Detox and Improve Yourself* for FREE here:

https://BookHip.com/LGQXHHH

PART FOUR

DR. SEBI JOURNAL

30 DAYS TO DETOX AND IMPROVE YOURSELF. IN THIS MOTIVATION JOURNAL BASED ON DR. SEBI'S PLANT-BASED ALKALINE DIET, YOU CAN KEEP TRACK OF YOUR MEALS, GOALS, AND PROGRESS.

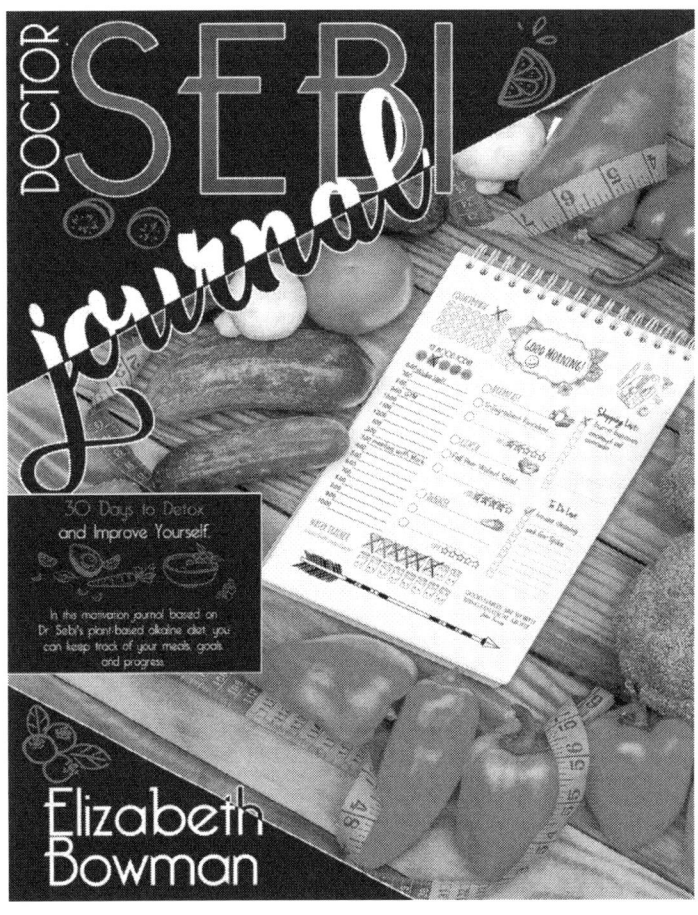

STICK IT ON THE FRIDGE!

NUTRITIONAL GUIDE

- If a food is not listed in this Nutritional Guide, it is NOT recommended.
- Drink one gallon of natural spring water daily.
- Take Dr. Sebi's products one hour before pharmaceuticals.
- All of Dr. Sebi's products may be taken together with no interaction.
- Following the Nutritional Guide strictly and taking the products regularly produces the best results with reversing disease.
- No animal products, no dairy, no fish, no hybrid foods and no alcohol.
- Natural growing grains are alkaline-based; it is recommended that you consume only the grains listed in the Nutritional Guide instead of wheat.
- Many of the grains listed in the Nutritional Guide are available as pasta, bread, flour or cereal and can be purchased at better health food stores.
- Dr. Sebi's products are still releasing therapeutic properties 14 days after being taken.
- Dr. Sebi says, *"Avoid using a microwave, it will kill your food."*
- Dr. Sebi says, *"No canned or seedless fruits"*

Vegetables

- Amaranth greens (Callaloo, a variety of greens)
- Avocado
- Bell Peppers
- Chayote (Mexican squash)
- Cucumber
- Dandelion greens
- Garbanzo beans
- Izote (Cactus flower/cactus leaf)
- Kale
- Lettuce (All, except Iceberg)
- Mushrooms (All, except Shitake)
- Nopales (Mexican cactus)
- Okra
- Olives
- Onions
- Sea Vegetables (Wakame/dulse/arame/hijiki/nori)
- Squash
- Tomato (Cherry and plum only)
- Tomatillo
- Turnip greens
- Zucchini
- Watercress
- Purslane (Verdolaga)
- Wild arugula

Natural Herbal Teas

- Burdock
- Chamomile
- Elderberry
- Fennel
- Ginger
- Raspberry
- Tila

Fruits

- Apples (Granny Smith and Red delicious not recommended)
- Bananas (The smallest one or the Burro/midsize/original banana)
- Berries (All varieties, no cranberries)
- Elderberries (In any form)
- Cantaloupe
- Cherries
- Currants
- Dates
- Figs
- Grapes (Seeded)
- Limes (Key limes, with seeds)

Grains

- Amaranth
- Fonio
- Kamut
- Quinoa
- Rye
- Spelt
- Tef
- Wild Rice

Nuts & Seeds

- Hemp Seeds
- Raw Sesame Seeds
- Raw Sesame "Tahini" Butter
- Walnuts
- Brazil Nuts

Oils

- Olive Oil (Do not cook)
- Coconut Oil (Do not cook)
- Grapeseed Oil
- Sesame Oil
- Hempseed Oil
- Avocado Oil

Mild Flavors

- Basil
- Bay Leaf
- Cloves
- Dill
- Oregano
- Savory
- Sweet Basil
- Tarragon
- Thyme

Pungent and Spicy Flavors

- Achiote
- Cayenne/ African Bird Pepper
- Coriander (Cilantro)
- Onion Powder
- Habanero
- Sage

Salty Flavors

- Pure Sea Salt
- Powdered Granulated Seaweed
- (Kelp/Dulse/Nori – has "sea taste")

Sweet Flavors

- Pure Agave Syrup (From cactus)
- Date Sugar

HOW TO COMPILE THE "DETOX DAILY DIARY"

Compiling the journal in all parts is very important for your physical and mental development. Keeping track of your thoughts, progress, and even your delusions will help you understand your self's changes.

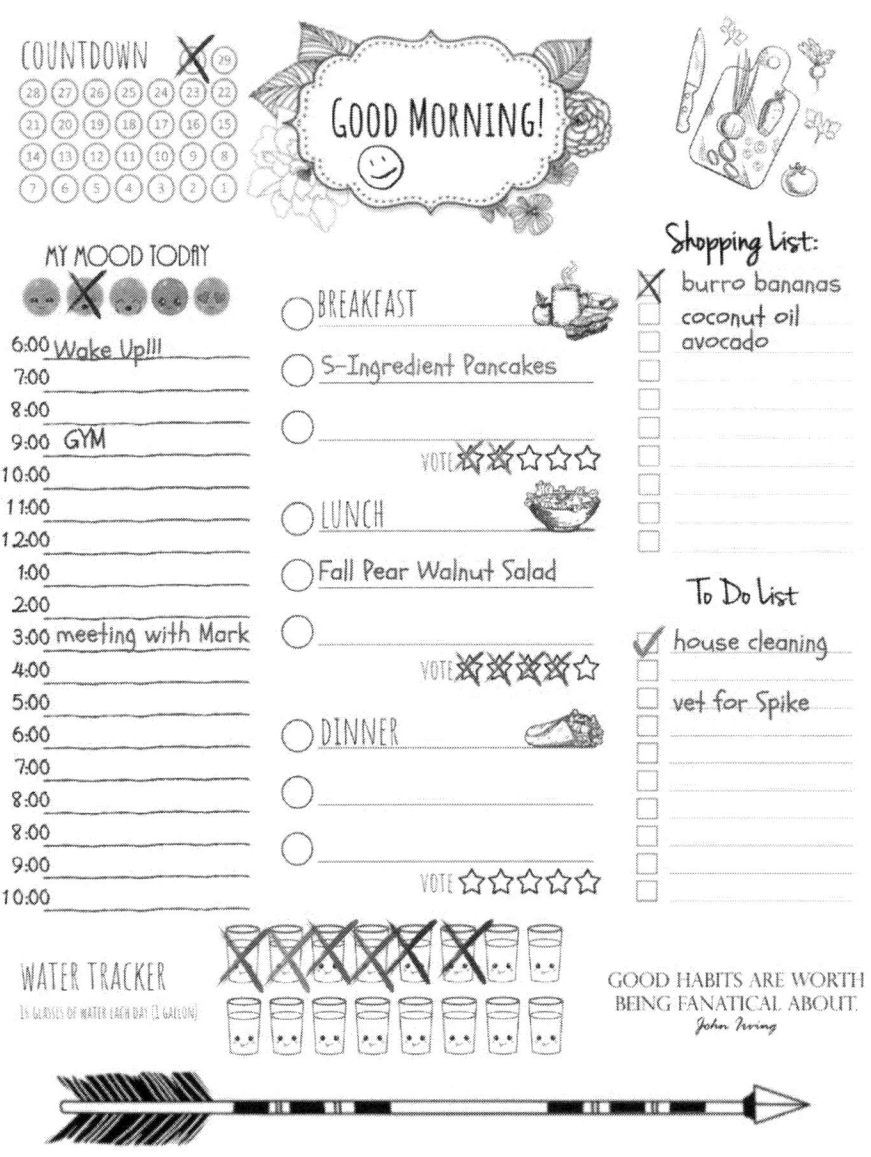

DAILY DIARY INSTRUCTIONS

COUNTDOWN

As you begin your journey the 30-day countdown to complete detoxification will begin.

You can use this "undated daily planner" at any point of the year.

SHOPPING LIST

in this section, you can write down all the ingredients you will need to prepare the day's meals and compile a shopping list.

MEAL PLANNER

Use this space to plan or log your daily meals and snacks easily

VOTE

Rate your recipes

NOTES

write the negative and positive aspects of the day

WATER TRACKER

Drinking water is essential!

Keep track of every glass of water you drink.

16 glasses of water = 1 gallon = 3.8 liters

TO DO LIST

Think about your intentions for today and tomorrow, note them down so you don't forget anything

CITATIONS

Here you will find some quotes that will help you in your journey

WEEKLY RESULTS INSTRUCTIONS

At the end of each week record all your progress on the physical and mental detox plan.

Check and track your weight.

Think about the past week, identify your goals, and analyze the behaviors that you can improve.

Target your priorities for the following week.

MONTHLY RESULTS INSTRUCTIONS

At the end of 30 days you will have completed your detoxification program.

Check and track your weight.

Review the past month and record your goals.

Compare your results with the information that you wrote on the "presentation page" 30 days ago.

Only in this way will you be able to understand the real benefits you have

achieved for your physical and mental health.

HOW TO PRINT THE PLANNER

You can either print directly by clicking on the printer icon or save the planner on your PC and print from the file..

When printing directly from the app, check the print preview before you print. If the printable does not fit on the page then change the settings until it does fit (for example, click on "fit on page" if your browser has that option).

Alternatively, just download the file and open it to print.

If you cannot print directly (for example if you have a popup blocker installed on your PC) then just download the file and print from your PC.

LET'S GO !!!

NAME _____

GENDER _____

AGE _____

HEIGHT _____

WEIGHT _____

0%

PHYSICAL DISEASES

☐ _____
☐ _____
☐ _____
☐ _____
☐ _____
☐ _____
☐ _____
☐ _____

WHAT ARE YOUR GOALS? WHAT WOULD YOU LIKE TO IMPROVE?

MIND   **BODY**

_____
_____
_____
_____

SUNDAY	MONDAY	TUESDAY	WEDNESDAY	THURSDAY	FRIDAY	SATURDAY	NOTES

0 1 2 3 4 5 6 7
8 9 10 11 12 13 14 15
16 17 18 19 20 21 22 23
24 25 26 27 28 29 30

Stay **determined**

COUNTDOWN

30 29 28 27 26 25 24 23 22 21 20 19 18 17 16 15 14 13 12 11 10 9 8 7 6 5 4 3 2 1

Good Morning!

MY MOOD TODAY

6:00
7:00
8:00
9:00
10:00
11:00
12:00
1:00
2:00
3:00
4:00
5:00
6:00
7:00
8:00
8:00
9:00
10:00

○ BREAKFAST

VOTE ☆☆☆☆☆

○ LUNCH

VOTE ☆☆☆☆☆

○ DINNER

VOTE ☆☆☆☆☆

Shopping List:

To Do list

WATER TRACKER
16 GLASSES OF WATER EACH DAY (1 GALLON)

GOOD HABITS ARE WORTH BEING FANATICAL ABOUT.
John Irving

COUNTDOWN

30 29 28 27 26 25 24 23 22 21 20 19 18 17 16 15 14 13 12 11 10 9 8 7 6 5 4 3 2 1

Good Morning!

MY MOOD TODAY

6:00
7:00
8:00
9:00
10:00
11:00
12:00
1:00
2:00
3:00
4:00
5:00
6:00
7:00
8:00
8:00
9:00
10:00

○ BREAKFAST

VOTE ☆☆☆☆☆

○ LUNCH

VOTE ☆☆☆☆☆

○ DINNER

VOTE ☆☆☆☆☆

Shopping List:

To Do List

The greatest pleasure in life is doing what people say you cannot do.

Walter Bagehot

WATER TRACKER
16 glasses of water each day (1 gallon)

COUNTDOWN

30 29 28 27 26 25 24 23 22 21 20 19 18 17 16 15 14 13 12 11 10 9 8 7 6 5 4 3 2 1

Good Morning!

MY MOOD TODAY

6:00
7:00
8:00
9:00
10:00
11:00
12:00
1:00
2:00
3:00
4:00
5:00
6:00
7:00
8:00
8:00
9:00
10:00

○ BREAKFAST

○
○
○

VOTE ☆☆☆☆☆

○ LUNCH

○
○
○

VOTE ☆☆☆☆☆

○ DINNER

○
○

VOTE ☆☆☆☆☆

Shopping List:

To Do List

WATER TRACKER
16 glasses of water each day (1 gallon)

DON'T expect to see a **CHANGE** if **YOU DON'T** *make one*

COUNTDOWN

30, 29, 28, 27, 26, 25, 24, 23, 22, 21, 20, 19, 18, 17, 16, 15, 14, 13, 12, 11, 10, 9, 8, 7, 6, 5, 4, 3, 2, 1

Good Morning!

MY MOOD TODAY

6:00	
7:00	
8:00	
9:00	
10:00	
11:00	
12:00	
1:00	
2:00	
3:00	
4:00	
5:00	
6:00	
7:00	
8:00	
8:00	
9:00	
10:00	

○ BREAKFAST

○ _____

○ _____

VOTE ☆☆☆☆☆

○ LUNCH

○ _____

○ _____

VOTE ☆☆☆☆☆

○ DINNER

○ _____

○ _____

VOTE ☆☆☆☆☆

WATER TRACKER
16 glasses of water each day (1 gallon)

Shopping List:
☐
☐
☐
☐
☐
☐
☐
☐
☐
☐

To Do List
☐
☐
☐
☐
☐
☐
☐
☐
☐
☐

THE FIRST STEP TO GETTING ANYWHERE IS DECIDING THAT YOU NO LONGER WANT TO STAY WHERE YOU ARE.

COUNTDOWN

30, 29, 28, 27, 26, 25, 24, 23, 22, 21, 20, 19, 18, 17, 16, 15, 14, 13, 12, 11, 10, 9, 8, 7, 6, 5, 4, 3, 2, 1

Good Morning!

MY MOOD TODAY

- 6:00
- 7:00
- 8:00
- 9:00
- 10:00
- 11:00
- 12:00
- 1:00
- 2:00
- 3:00
- 4:00
- 5:00
- 6:00
- 7:00
- 8:00
- 8:00
- 9:00
- 10:00

○ BREAKFAST

○

○

VOTE ☆☆☆☆☆

○ LUNCH

○

○

VOTE ☆☆☆☆☆

○ DINNER

○

○

VOTE ☆☆☆☆☆

Shopping List:

To Do List

WATER TRACKER
16 GLASSES OF WATER EACH DAY (1 GALLON)

> Do what you **have to do** *until* you can do what you **want to do**
>
> Oprah Winfrey

COUNTDOWN

30 29 28 27 26 25 24 23 22 21 20 19 18 17 16 15 14 13 12 11 10 9 8 7 6 5 4 3 2 1

Good Morning!

MY MOOD TODAY

6:00
7:00
8:00
9:00
10:00
11:00
12:00
1:00
2:00
3:00
4:00
5:00
6:00
7:00
8:00
8:00
9:00
10:00

○ BREAKFAST

VOTE ☆☆☆☆☆

○ LUNCH

VOTE ☆☆☆☆☆

○ DINNER

VOTE ☆☆☆☆☆

Shopping List:

To Do List

WATER TRACKER
16 GLASSES OF WATER EACH DAY (1 GALLON)

YOU ONLY fail when you STOP trying

COUNTDOWN

30 29 28 27 26 25 24 23 22 21 20 19 18 17 16 15 14 13 12 11 10 9 8 7 6 5 4 3 2 1

Good Morning!

MY MOOD TODAY

6:00
7:00
8:00
9:00
10:00
11:00
12:00
1:00
2:00
3:00
4:00
5:00
6:00
7:00
8:00
8:00
9:00
10:00

○ BREAKFAST

VOTE ☆☆☆☆☆

○ LUNCH

VOTE ☆☆☆☆☆

○ DINNER

VOTE ☆☆☆☆☆

Shopping List:

To Do list

LIVE AS IF YOU WERE TO DIE TOMORROW. LEARN AS IF YOU WERE TO LIVE FOREVER.

Mahatma Gandhi

WATER TRACKER
16 GLASSES OF WATER EACH DAY (1 GALLON)

WEEKLY RESULTS

WEEK 1 2 3 4

WEIGHT _____

LOST WEIGHT _____

25%

WEEKLY GOALS

○ _____
○ _____
○ _____

Check your goals for the past week. Are you satisfied? Give yourself an honest rating on a scale of 1 to 10

_____
_____
_____

What did you do and what could you better?

_____
_____
_____
_____

- FOR THE NEXT WEEK -

TO DO LIST
☐ _____
☐ _____
☐ _____
☐ _____
☐ _____
☐ _____
☐ _____
☐ _____
☐ _____

NOTES
_____
_____
_____
_____
_____
_____
_____

TOP 3 PRIORITIES
○ _____
○ _____
○ _____

YOU ONLY fail when you STOP trying

COUNTDOWN

30 29 28 27 26 25 24 23 22 21 20 19 18 17 16 15 14 13 12 11 10 9 8 7 6 5 4 3 2 1

Good Morning!

MY MOOD TODAY

- 6:00
- 7:00
- 8:00
- 9:00
- 10:00
- 11:00
- 12:00
- 1:00
- 2:00
- 3:00
- 4:00
- 5:00
- 6:00
- 7:00
- 8:00
- 8:00
- 9:00
- 10:00

○ BREAKFAST

VOTE ☆☆☆☆☆

○ LUNCH

VOTE ☆☆☆☆☆

○ DINNER

VOTE ☆☆☆☆☆

Shopping List:

To Do List

Life isn't about finding yourself. Life is about creating yourself.

— George Bernard Shaw

WATER TRACKER
16 GLASSES OF WATER EACH DAY (1 GALLON)

COUNTDOWN

30 29 28 27 26 25 24 23 22 21 20 19 18 17 16 15 14 13 12 11 10 9 8 7 6 5 4 3 2 1

Good Morning!

MY MOOD TODAY

6:00
7:00
8:00
9:00
10:00
11:00
12:00
1:00
2:00
3:00
4:00
5:00
6:00
7:00
8:00
8:00
9:00
10:00

○ BREAKFAST

VOTE ☆☆☆☆☆

○ LUNCH

VOTE ☆☆☆☆☆

○ DINNER

VOTE ☆☆☆☆☆

Shopping List:

To Do List

WATER TRACKER
16 GLASSES OF WATER EACH DAY (1 GALLON)

Be stronger than your excuses

COUNTDOWN

30 29 28 27 26 25 24 23 22 21 20 19 18 17 16 15 14 13 12 11 10 9 8 7 6 5 4 3 2 1

Good Morning!

MY MOOD TODAY

6:00
7:00
8:00
9:00
10:00
11:00
12:00
1:00
2:00
3:00
4:00
5:00
6:00
7:00
8:00
8:00
9:00
10:00

○ BREAKFAST

VOTE ☆☆☆☆☆

○ LUNCH

VOTE ☆☆☆☆☆

○ DINNER

VOTE ☆☆☆☆☆

Shopping List:

To Do List

WATER TRACKER
16 GLASSES OF WATER EACH DAY (1 GALLON)

LIFE BEGINS AT THE END OF YOUR COMFORT ZONE.

Good Morning!

COUNTDOWN
30, 29, 28, 27, 26, 25, 24, 23, 22, 21, 20, 19, 18, 17, 16, 15, 14, 13, 12, 11, 10, 9, 8, 7, 6, 5, 4, 3, 2, 1

MY MOOD TODAY

- 6:00
- 7:00
- 8:00
- 9:00
- 10:00
- 11:00
- 12:00
- 1:00
- 2:00
- 3:00
- 4:00
- 5:00
- 6:00
- 7:00
- 8:00
- 8:00
- 9:00
- 10:00

○ BREAKFAST
_____
_____
_____
VOTE ☆☆☆☆☆

○ LUNCH
_____
_____
_____
VOTE ☆☆☆☆☆

○ DINNER
_____
_____
_____
VOTE ☆☆☆☆☆

Shopping List:

To Do List

WATER TRACKER
16 GLASSES OF WATER EACH DAY (1 GALLON)

Don't STOP UNTIL you're PROUD

COUNTDOWN

30 29 28 27 26 25 24 23 22 21 20 19 18 17 16 15 14 13 12 11 10 9 8 7 6 5 4 3 2 1

Good Morning!

MY MOOD TODAY

6:00
7:00
8:00
9:00
10:00
11:00
12:00
1:00
2:00
3:00
4:00
5:00
6:00
7:00
8:00
8:00
9:00
10:00

○ BREAKFAST

VOTE ☆☆☆☆☆

○ LUNCH

VOTE ☆☆☆☆☆

○ DINNER

VOTE ☆☆☆☆☆

Shopping List:

To Do List

Knowing is not enough, we must apply. Willing is not enough, we must do.

Bruce Lee

WATER TRACKER
16 glasses of water each day (1 gallon)

Good Morning!

COUNTDOWN
30, 29, 28, 27, 26, 25, 24, 23, 22, 21, 20, 19, 18, 17, 16, 15, 14, 13, 12, 11, 10, 9, 8, 7, 6, 5, 4, 3, 2, 1

MY MOOD TODAY

6:00	
7:00	
8:00	
9:00	
10:00	
11:00	
12:00	
1:00	
2:00	
3:00	
4:00	
5:00	
6:00	
7:00	
8:00	
8:00	
9:00	
10:00	

BREAKFAST
VOTE ☆☆☆☆☆

LUNCH
VOTE ☆☆☆☆☆

DINNER
VOTE ☆☆☆☆☆

Shopping List:

To Do List

WATER TRACKER
16 GLASSES OF WATER EACH DAY (1 GALLON)

Great things NEVER came from Comfort zones

COUNTDOWN

30 29 28 27 26 25 24 23 22 21 20 19 18 17 16 15 14 13 12 11 10 9 8 7 6 5 4 3 2 1

Good Morning!

MY MOOD TODAY

- 6:00
- 7:00
- 8:00
- 9:00
- 10:00
- 11:00
- 12:00
- 1:00
- 2:00
- 3:00
- 4:00
- 5:00
- 6:00
- 7:00
- 8:00
- 8:00
- 9:00
- 10:00

○ BREAKFAST

○ ....

○ ....

VOTE ☆☆☆☆☆

○ LUNCH

○ ....

○ ....

VOTE ☆☆☆☆☆

○ DINNER

○ ....

○ ....

VOTE ☆☆☆☆☆

Shopping List:

To Do List

WATER TRACKER
16 GLASSES OF WATER EACH DAY (1 GALLON)

I can and I will WATCH ME

WEEKLY RESULTS

WEEK 1 2 3 4

WEIGHT _____

LOST WEIGHT _____

50%

WEEKLY GOALS
○ _____
○ _____
○ _____

Check your goals for the past week. Are you satisfied? Give yourself an honest rating on a scale of 1 to 10.

_____
_____
_____

What did you do and what could you better?

_____
_____
_____

— FOR THE NEXT WEEK —

TO DO LIST
☐ _____
☐ _____
☐ _____
☐ _____
☐ _____
☐ _____
☐ _____
☐ _____
☐ _____

NOTES
_____
_____
_____
_____
_____
_____
_____

TOP 3 PRIORITIES
○ _____
○ _____
○ _____

Great things never came from Comfort zones

COUNTDOWN

30 29 28 27 26 25 24 23 22 21 20 19 18 17 16 15 14 13 12 11 10 9 8 7 6 5 4 3 2 1

Good Morning!

MY MOOD TODAY

6:00
7:00
8:00
9:00
10:00
11:00
12:00
1:00
2:00
3:00
4:00
5:00
6:00
7:00
8:00
8:00
9:00
10:00

○ BREAKFAST

VOTE ☆☆☆☆☆

○ LUNCH

VOTE ☆☆☆☆☆

○ DINNER

VOTE ☆☆☆☆☆

Shopping List:

To Do List

IF YOU BELIEVE IN YOURSELF ANYTHING IS POSSIBLE.

WATER TRACKER
16 GLASSES OF WATER EACH DAY (1 GALLON)

COUNTDOWN

30 29 28 27 26 25 24 23 22 21 20 19 18 17 16 15 14 13 12 11 10 9 8 7 6 5 4 3 2 1

Good Morning!

MY MOOD TODAY

6:00	
7:00	
8:00	
9:00	
10:00	
11:00	
12:00	
1:00	
2:00	
3:00	
4:00	
5:00	
6:00	
7:00	
8:00	
8:00	
9:00	
10:00	

○ BREAKFAST

VOTE ☆☆☆☆☆

○ LUNCH

VOTE ☆☆☆☆☆

○ DINNER

VOTE ☆☆☆☆☆

Shopping List:

To Do List

Discipline is choosing between *what you want* NOW and *what you want* MOST
Abraham Lincoln

WATER TRACKER
15 GLASSES OF WATER EACH DAY (1 GALLON)

Good Morning!

COUNTDOWN
30, 29, 28, 27, 26, 25, 24, 23, 22, 21, 20, 19, 18, 17, 16, 15, 14, 13, 12, 11, 10, 9, 8, 7, 6, 5, 4, 3, 2, 1

MY MOOD TODAY

6:00	
7:00	
8:00	
9:00	
10:00	
11:00	
12:00	
1:00	
2:00	
3:00	
4:00	
5:00	
6:00	
7:00	
8:00	
8:00	
9:00	
10:00	

○ BREAKFAST
___
VOTE ☆☆☆☆☆

○ LUNCH
___
VOTE ☆☆☆☆☆

○ DINNER
___
VOTE ☆☆☆☆☆

Shopping list:

To Do list

IF IT IS IMPORTANT TO YOU, YOU WILL FIND A WAY. IF NOT, YOU WILL FIND AN EXCUSE.

Ryan Blair

WATER TRACKER
16 GLASSES OF WATER EACH DAY (1 GALLON)

COUNTDOWN

30 29 28 27 26 25 24 23 22 21 20 19 18 17 16 15 14 13 12 11 10 9 8 7 6 5 4 3 2 1

Good Morning!

MY MOOD TODAY

6:00
7:00
8:00
9:00
10:00
11:00
12:00
1:00
2:00
3:00
4:00
5:00
6:00
7:00
8:00
8:00
9:00
10:00

○ BREAKFAST
_____

○ _____

○ _____
VOTE ☆☆☆☆☆

○ LUNCH
_____

○ _____

○ _____
VOTE ☆☆☆☆☆

○ DINNER
_____

○ _____

○ _____
VOTE ☆☆☆☆☆

WATER TRACKER
16 GLASSES OF WATER EACH DAY (1 GALLON)

Shopping List:

To Do List

Do something **today** that your **future** *self* will **thank** you for

COUNTDOWN

30, 29, 28, 27, 26, 25, 24, 23, 22, 21, 20, 19, 18, 17, 16, 15, 14, 13, 12, 11, 10, 9, 8, 7, 6, 5, 4, 3, 2, 1

Good Morning!

MY MOOD TODAY

6:00
7:00
8:00
9:00
10:00
11:00
12:00
1:00
2:00
3:00
4:00
5:00
6:00
7:00
8:00
8:00
9:00
10:00

○ BREAKFAST

○
○
VOTE ☆☆☆☆☆

○ LUNCH

○
○
VOTE ☆☆☆☆☆

○ DINNER

○
○
VOTE ☆☆☆☆☆

Shopping List:

To Do List

I am not what happened to me, I am what I chose to become.

— Carl Jung

WATER TRACKER
16 GLASSES OF WATER EACH DAY (1 GALLON)

COUNTDOWN

30, 29, 28, 27, 26, 25, 24, 23, 22, 21, 20, 19, 18, 17, 16, 15, 14, 13, 12, 11, 10, 9, 8, 7, 6, 5, 4, 3, 2, 1

Good Morning!

MY MOOD TODAY

Schedule:
- 6:00
- 7:00
- 8:00
- 9:00
- 10:00
- 11:00
- 12:00
- 1:00
- 2:00
- 3:00
- 4:00
- 5:00
- 6:00
- 7:00
- 8:00
- 8:00
- 9:00
- 10:00

○ BREAKFAST

○
○

VOTE ☆☆☆☆☆

○ LUNCH

○
○

VOTE ☆☆☆☆☆

○ DINNER

○
○

VOTE ☆☆☆☆☆

Shopping list:

To Do list

WATER TRACKER
16 glasses of water each day (1 gallon)

Your are **What you do** *not* **what you say** you will do

COUNTDOWN

30 29 28 27 26 25 24 23 22 21 20 19 18 17 16 15 14 13 12 11 10 9 8 7 6 5 4 3 2 1

Good Morning!

MY MOOD TODAY

- 6:00
- 7:00
- 8:00
- 9:00
- 10:00
- 11:00
- 12:00
- 1:00
- 2:00
- 3:00
- 4:00
- 5:00
- 6:00
- 7:00
- 8:00
- 8:00
- 9:00
- 10:00

○ BREAKFAST

○

○

VOTE ☆☆☆☆☆

○ LUNCH

○

○

VOTE ☆☆☆☆☆

○ DINNER

○

○

VOTE ☆☆☆☆☆

Shopping List:

To Do List

Hard work beats talent when talent doesn't work hard.

— Tim Notke

WATER TRACKER
16 GLASSES OF WATER EACH DAY (1 GALLON)

WEEKLY RESULTS

WEEK [1] [2] [3] [4]

WEIGHT _____

LOST WEIGHT _____

75%

WEEKLY GOALS

○ _____
○ _____
○ _____

Check your goals for the past week. Are you satisfied? Give yourself an honest rating on a scale of 1 to 10.

_____
_____
_____

What did you do and what could you better?

_____
_____
_____

— FOR THE NEXT WEEK —

TO DO LIST
☐ _____
☐ _____
☐ _____
☐ _____
☐ _____
☐ _____
☐ _____
☐ _____
☐ _____

NOTES
_____
_____
_____
_____
_____
_____
_____

TOP 3 PRIORITIES
○ _____
○ _____
○ _____

LOVE THE LIFE YOU LIVE.
LIVE THE LIFE YOU LOVE.

Bob Marley

COUNTDOWN

30 29 28 27 26 25 24 23 22 21 20 19 18 17 16 15 14 13 12 11 10 9 8 7 6 5 4 3 2 1

Good Morning!

MY MOOD TODAY

6:00
7:00
8:00
9:00
10:00
11:00
12:00
1:00
2:00
3:00
4:00
5:00
6:00
7:00
8:00
8:00
9:00
10:00

○ BREAKFAST

○
○
VOTE ☆☆☆☆☆

○ LUNCH
○
○
VOTE ☆☆☆☆☆

○ DINNER
○
○
VOTE ☆☆☆☆☆

Shopping List:

To Do List

DOUBT KILLS MORE DREAMS THAN FAILURE EVER WILL.

Suzy Kassem

WATER TRACKER
16 GLASSES OF WATER EACH DAY (1 GALLON)

COUNTDOWN

30 29 28 27 26 25 24 23 22 21 20 19 18 17 16 15 14 13 12 11 10 9 8 7 6 5 4 3 2 1

Good Morning!

MY MOOD TODAY

6:00
7:00
8:00
9:00
10:00
11:00
12:00
1:00
2:00
3:00
4:00
5:00
6:00
7:00
8:00
8:00
9:00
10:00

○ BREAKFAST

VOTE ☆☆☆☆☆

○ LUNCH

VOTE ☆☆☆☆☆

○ DINNER

VOTE ☆☆☆☆☆

Shopping List:

To Do List

WATER TRACKER
16 GLASSES OF WATER EACH DAY (1 GALLON)

DON'T STOP WHEN YOU ARE TIRED. STOP WHEN YOU ARE DONE.

COUNTDOWN

30, 29, 28, 27, 26, 25, 24, 23, 22, 21, 20, 19, 18, 17, 16, 15, 14, 13, 12, 11, 10, 9, 8, 7, 6, 5, 4, 3, 2, 1

Good Morning!

MY MOOD TODAY

6:00
7:00
8:00
9:00
10:00
11:00
12:00
1:00
2:00
3:00
4:00
5:00
6:00
7:00
8:00
8:00
9:00
10:00

○ BREAKFAST

○ _____

○ _____

VOTE ☆☆☆☆☆

○ LUNCH

○ _____

○ _____

VOTE ☆☆☆☆☆

○ DINNER

○ _____

○ _____

VOTE ☆☆☆☆☆

Shopping List:

☐
☐
☐
☐
☐
☐
☐
☐
☐
☐

To Do List

☐
☐
☐
☐
☐
☐
☐
☐
☐
☐

WATER TRACKER
16 GLASSES OF WATER EACH DAY (1 GALLON)

A Negative mind will NEVER give you a Positive life

Good Morning!

COUNTDOWN

30, 29, 28, 27, 26, 25, 24, 23, 22, 21, 20, 19, 18, 17, 16, 15, 14, 13, 12, 11, 10, 9, 8, 7, 6, 5, 4, 3, 2, 1

MY MOOD TODAY

6:00	
7:00	
8:00	
9:00	
10:00	
11:00	
12:00	
1:00	
2:00	
3:00	
4:00	
5:00	
6:00	
7:00	
8:00	
8:00	
9:00	
10:00	

○ BREAKFAST

○ _____

○ _____

VOTE ☆☆☆☆☆

○ LUNCH

○ _____

○ _____

VOTE ☆☆☆☆☆

○ DINNER

○ _____

○ _____

VOTE ☆☆☆☆☆

Shopping List:

To Do List

WATER TRACKER
16 GLASSES OF WATER EACH DAY (1 GALLON)

DIFFICULT ROADS OFTEN LEAD TO BEAUTIFUL DESTINATIONS.

COUNTDOWN

30 29 28 27 26 25 24 23 22 21 20 19 18 17 16 15 14 13 12 11 10 9 8 7 6 5 4 3 2 1

Good Morning!

MY MOOD TODAY

6:00
7:00
8:00
9:00
10:00
11:00
12:00
1:00
2:00
3:00
4:00
5:00
6:00
7:00
8:00
8:00
9:00
10:00

○ BREAKFAST

○
○
VOTE ☆☆☆☆☆

○ LUNCH

○
○
VOTE ☆☆☆☆☆

○ DINNER

○
○
VOTE ☆☆☆☆☆

Shopping List:

To Do List

A RIVER CUTS THROUGH ROCK, NOT BECAUSE OF ITS POWER, BUT BECAUSE OF ITS PERSISTENCE.

Jim Watkins

WATER TRACKER
16 GLASSES OF WATER EACH DAY (1 GALLON)

COUNTDOWN

30 29 28 27 26 25 24 23 22 21 20 19 18 17 16 15 14 13 12 11 10 9 8 7 6 5 4 3 2 1

Good Morning!

MY MOOD TODAY

6:00
7:00
8:00
9:00
10:00
11:00
12:00
1:00
2:00
3:00
4:00
5:00
6:00
7:00
8:00
8:00
9:00
10:00

○ BREAKFAST

VOTE ☆☆☆☆☆

○ LUNCH

VOTE ☆☆☆☆☆

○ DINNER

VOTE ☆☆☆☆☆

Shopping List:

To Do List

WATER TRACKER
16 GLASSES OF WATER EACH DAY (1 GALLON)

Motivation is what gets you started.
Habit is what keeps you going.
Jim Rohn

COUNTDOWN

30 29 28 27 26 25 24 23 22 21 20 19 18 17 16 15 14 13 12 11 10 9 8 7 6 5 4 3 2 1

Good Morning!

MY MOOD TODAY

6:00
7:00
8:00
9:00
10:00
11:00
12:00
1:00
2:00
3:00
4:00
5:00
6:00
7:00
8:00
8:00
9:00
10:00

○ BREAKFAST

VOTE ☆☆☆☆☆

○ LUNCH

VOTE ☆☆☆☆☆

○ DINNER

VOTE ☆☆☆☆☆

Shopping List:

To Do List

INHALE
love
EXHALE
gratitude

WATER TRACKER
16 GLASSES OF WATER EACH DAY (1 GALLON)

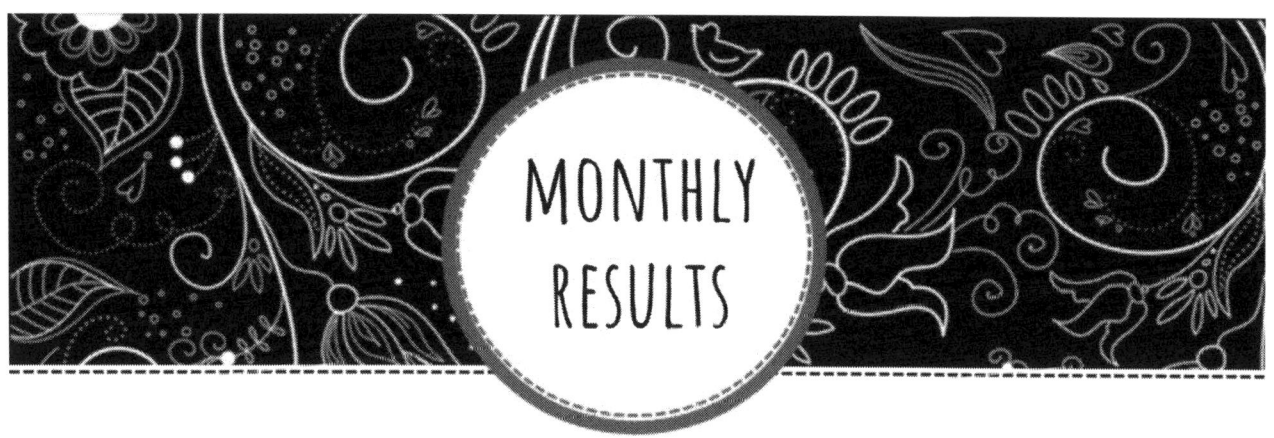

MONTHLY RESULTS

CONGRATULATIONS, YOU HAVE COMPLETED YOUR DEXOTIFICATION JOURNEY!

WEIGHT _____

LOST WEIGHT _____

100%

MONTHLY GOALS
○ _____
○ _____
○ _____

HOW DO YOU FEEL ABOUT YOUR PHYSICAL AND MENTAL STATE NOW?

_____
_____
_____

COMPARE YOUR ANSWER TO THE GOALS YOU WROTE A MONTH AGO.
ARE YOU SATISFIED WITH YOUR RESULTS?

_____
_____
_____

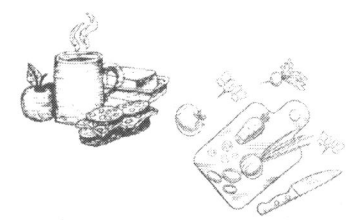

Results can only change when we change our consistent actions and make them habits.
Billy Cox

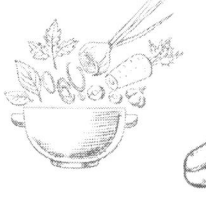
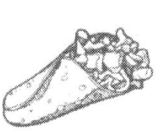
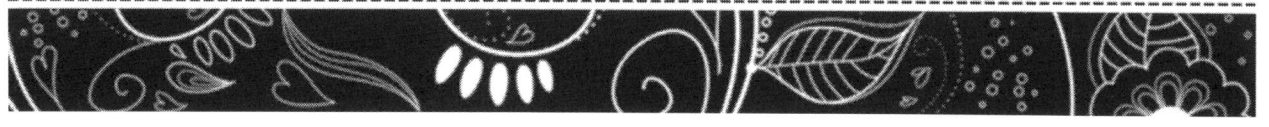

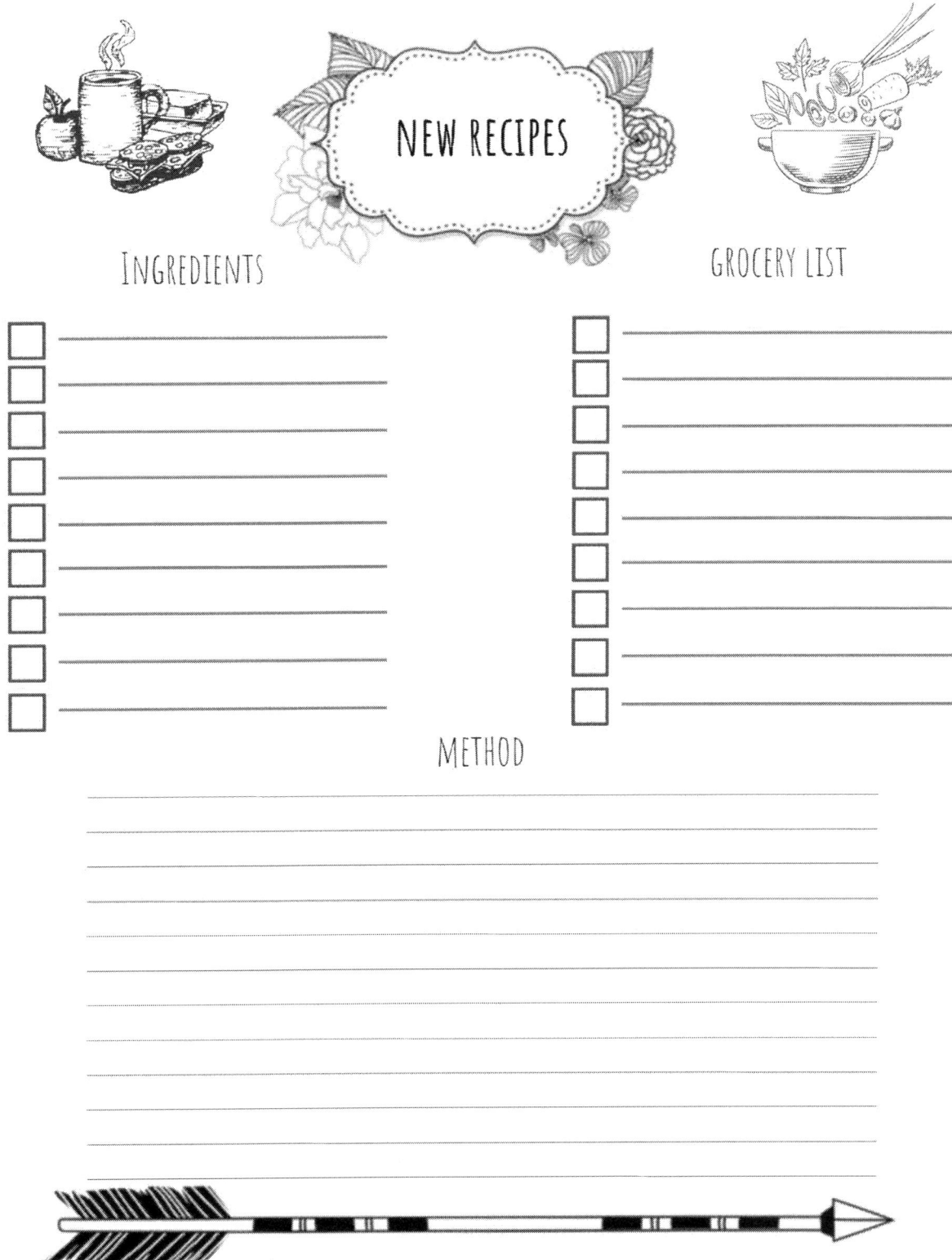

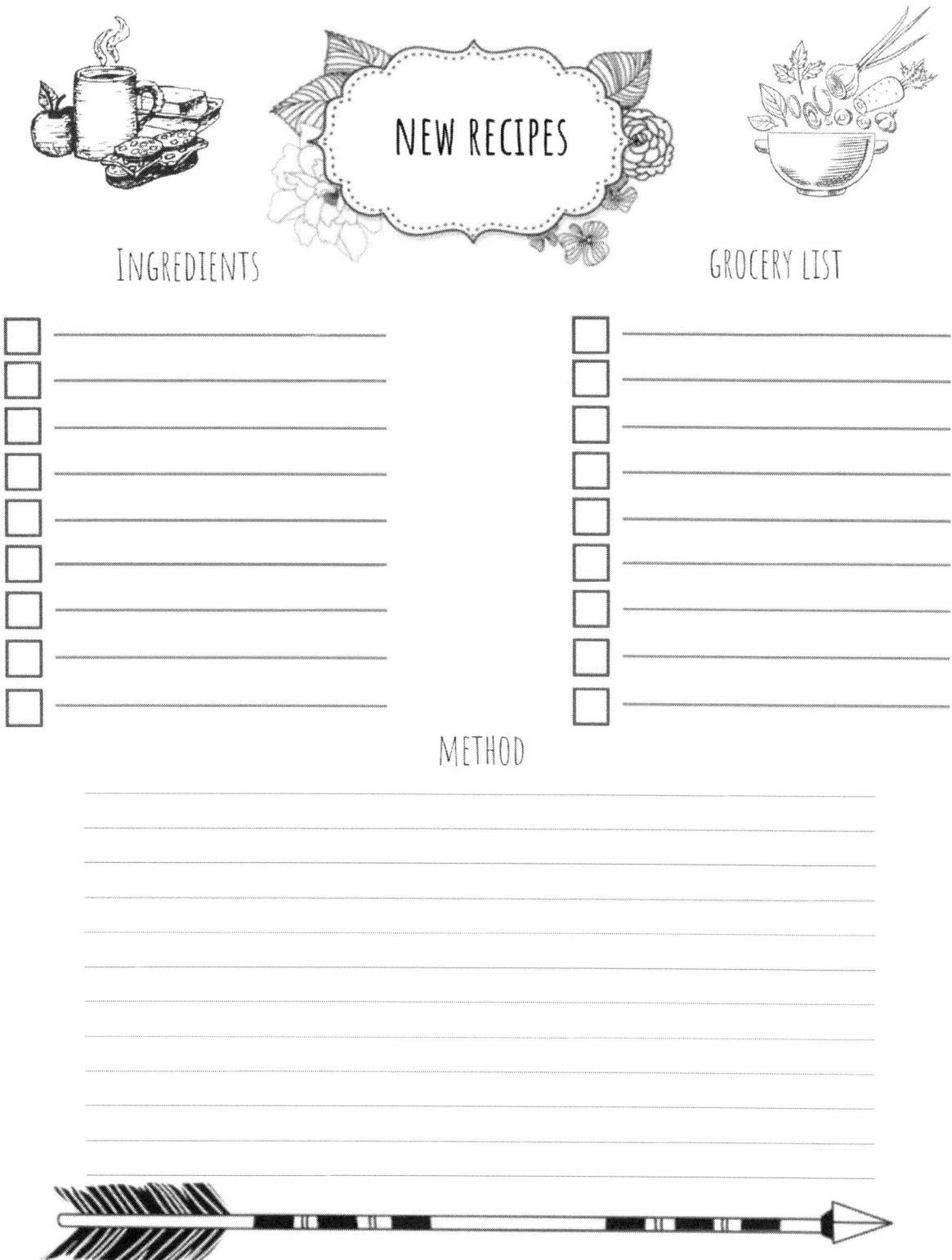

NEW RECIPES

Ingredients

- [ ] _____
- [ ] _____
- [ ] _____
- [ ] _____
- [ ] _____
- [ ] _____
- [ ] _____
- [ ] _____
- [ ] _____

Grocery List

- [ ] _____
- [ ] _____
- [ ] _____
- [ ] _____
- [ ] _____
- [ ] _____
- [ ] _____
- [ ] _____
- [ ] _____

Method

_____
_____
_____
_____
_____
_____
_____
_____
_____
_____

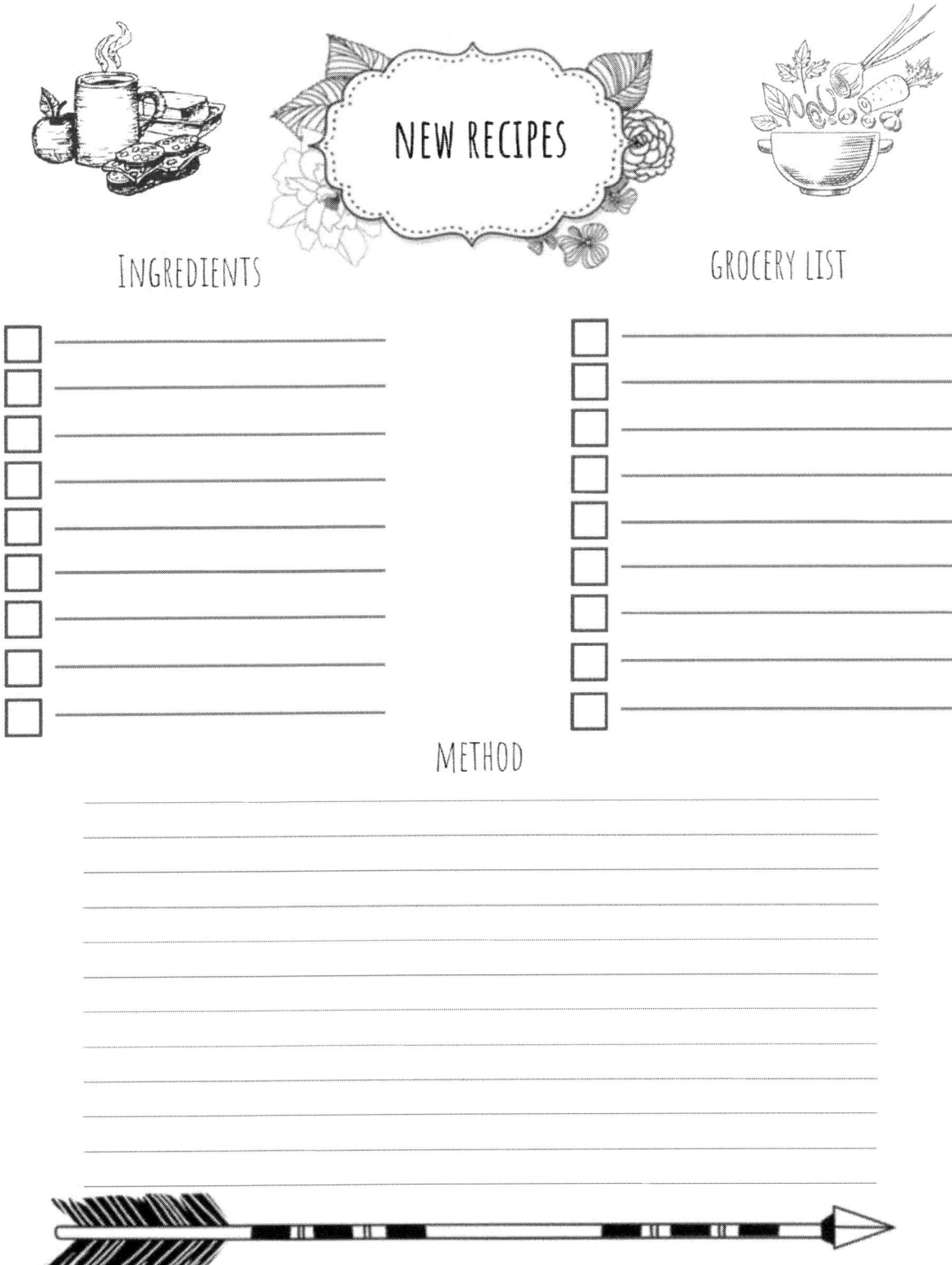

NEW RECIPES

Ingredients
- [ ]
- [ ]
- [ ]
- [ ]
- [ ]
- [ ]
- [ ]
- [ ]
- [ ]

Grocery List
- [ ]
- [ ]
- [ ]
- [ ]
- [ ]
- [ ]
- [ ]
- [ ]
- [ ]

Method

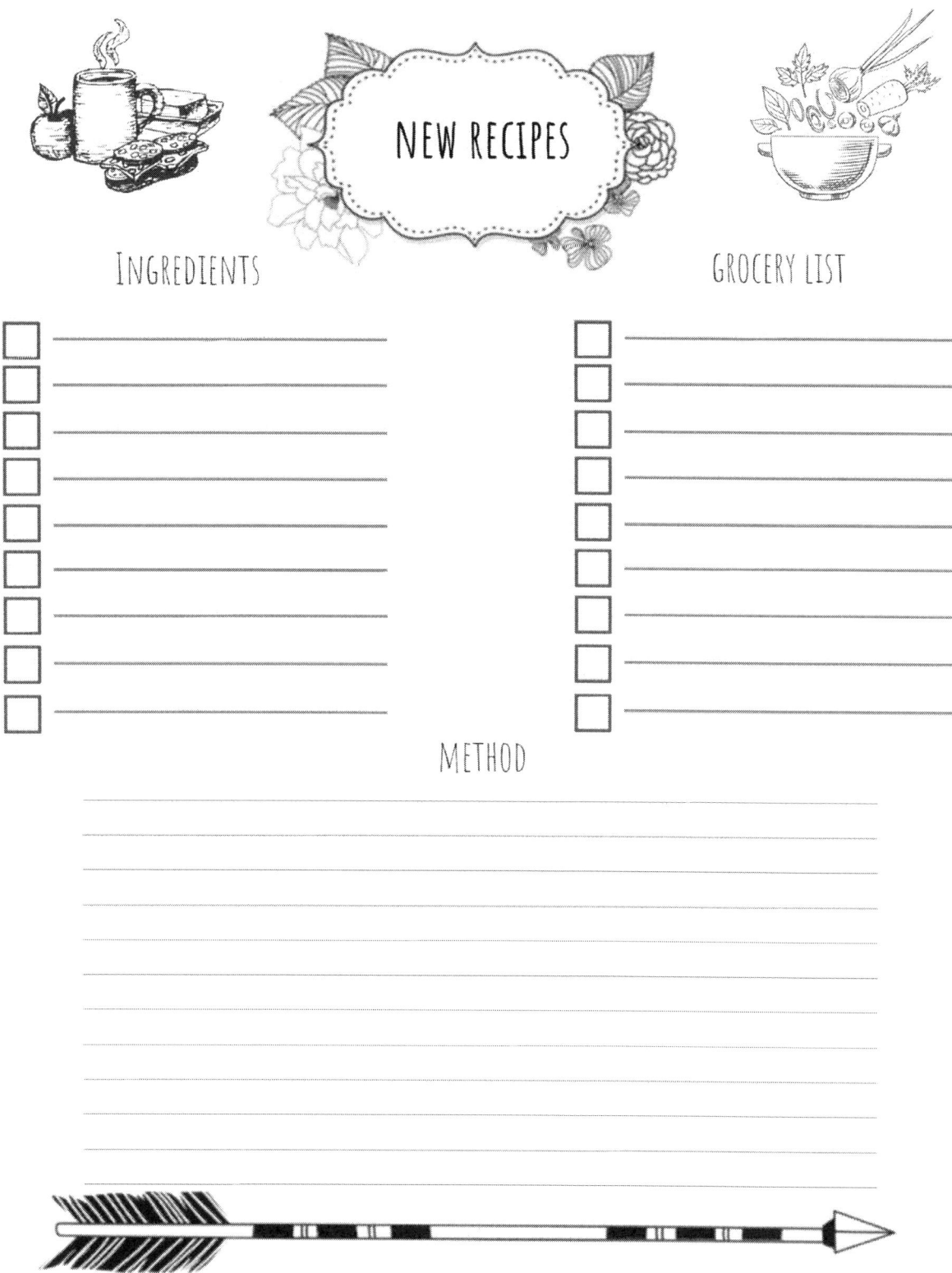

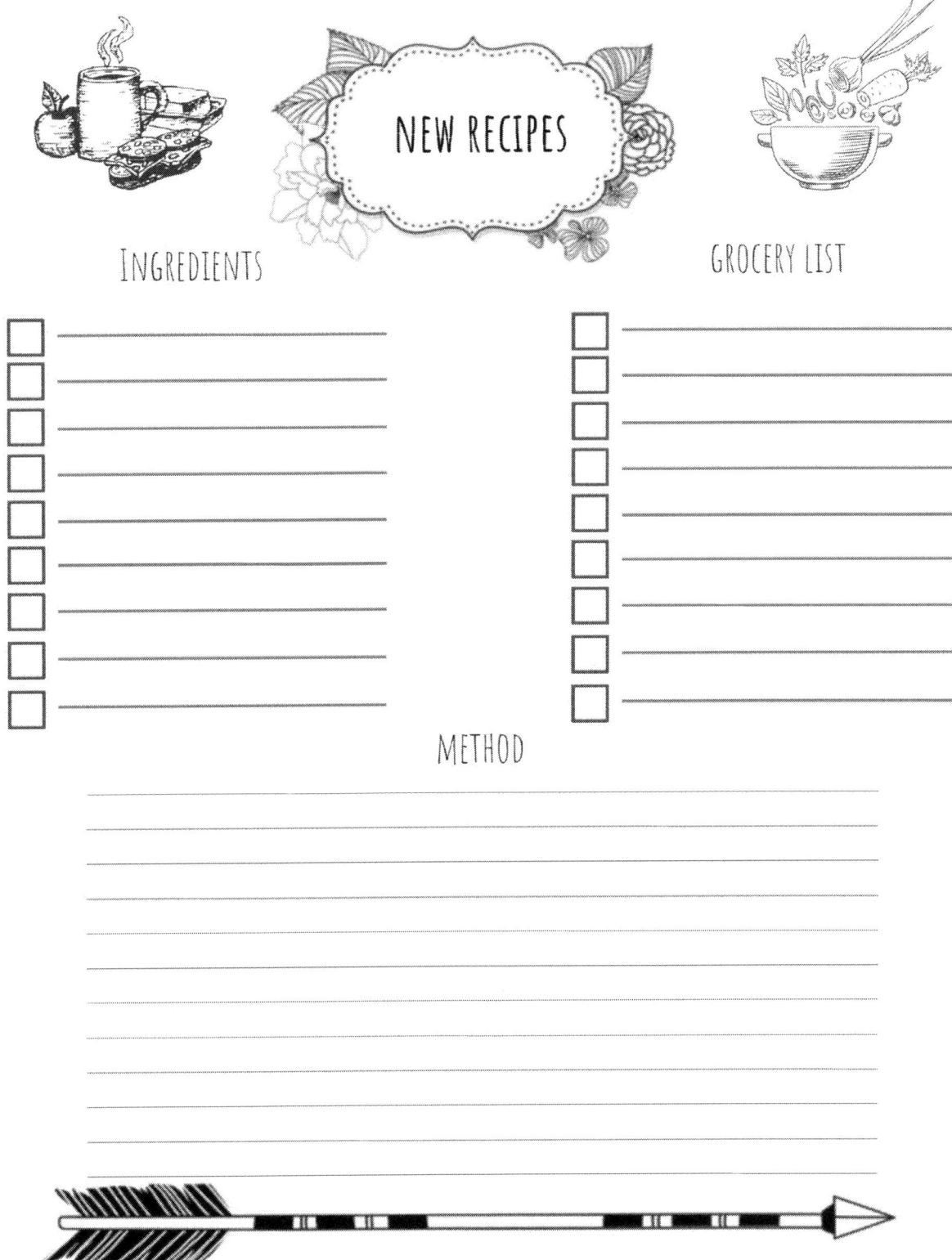

NEW RECIPES

INGREDIENTS

- [ ] _____
- [ ] _____
- [ ] _____
- [ ] _____
- [ ] _____
- [ ] _____
- [ ] _____
- [ ] _____
- [ ] _____

GROCERY LIST

- [ ] _____
- [ ] _____
- [ ] _____
- [ ] _____
- [ ] _____
- [ ] _____
- [ ] _____
- [ ] _____
- [ ] _____

METHOD

_____
_____
_____
_____
_____
_____
_____
_____
_____
_____

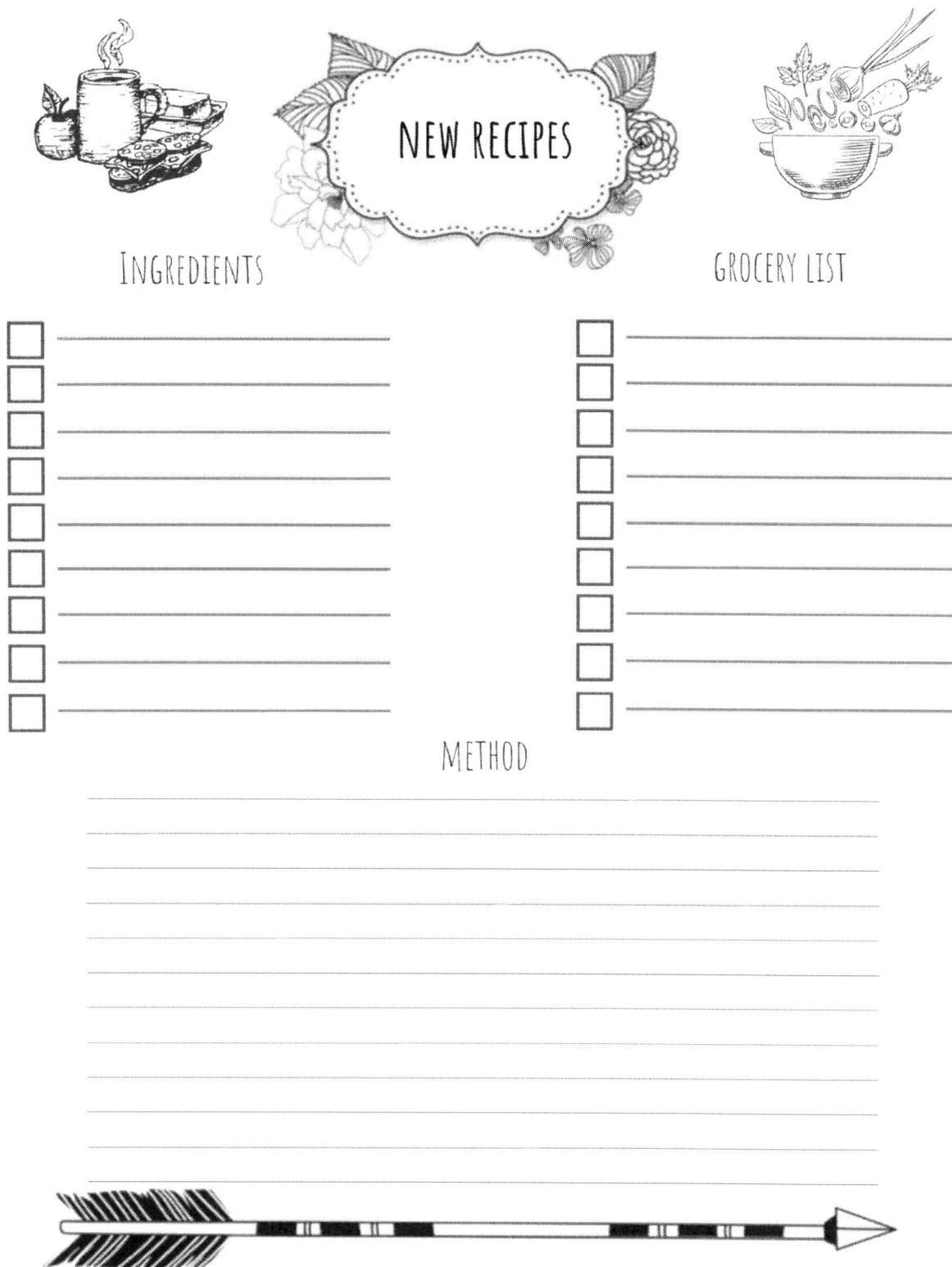

NEW RECIPES

Ingredients

- [ ] _____
- [ ] _____
- [ ] _____
- [ ] _____
- [ ] _____
- [ ] _____
- [ ] _____
- [ ] _____
- [ ] _____

Grocery List

- [ ] _____
- [ ] _____
- [ ] _____
- [ ] _____
- [ ] _____
- [ ] _____
- [ ] _____
- [ ] _____
- [ ] _____

Method

_____
_____
_____
_____
_____
_____
_____
_____
_____
_____

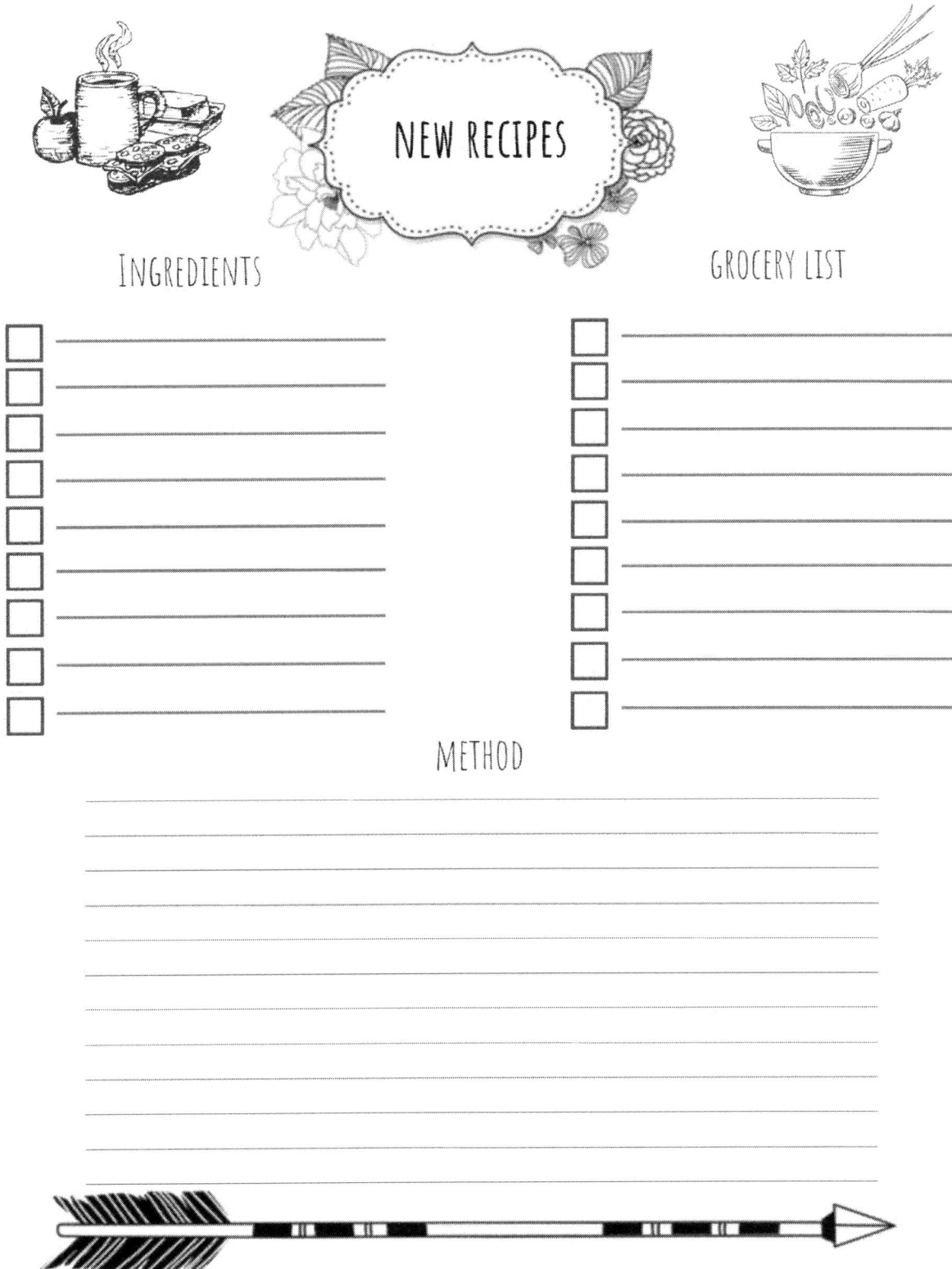

NEW RECIPES

INGREDIENTS

- [ ]
- [ ]
- [ ]
- [ ]
- [ ]
- [ ]
- [ ]
- [ ]
- [ ]

GROCERY LIST

- [ ]
- [ ]
- [ ]
- [ ]
- [ ]
- [ ]
- [ ]
- [ ]
- [ ]

METHOD

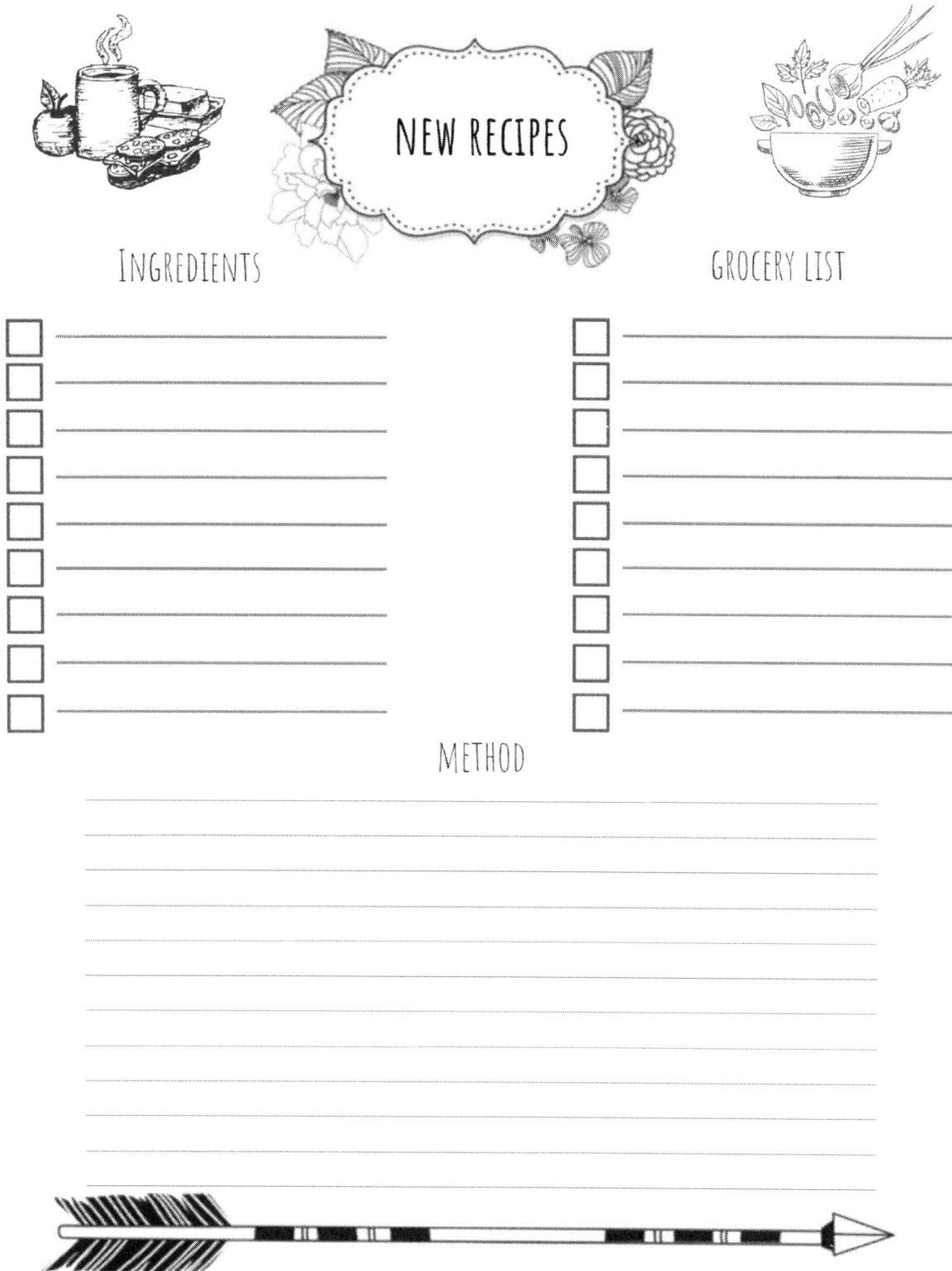

NEW RECIPES

INGREDIENTS

- [ ]
- [ ]
- [ ]
- [ ]
- [ ]
- [ ]
- [ ]
- [ ]
- [ ]

GROCERY LIST

- [ ]
- [ ]
- [ ]
- [ ]
- [ ]
- [ ]
- [ ]
- [ ]
- [ ]

METHOD

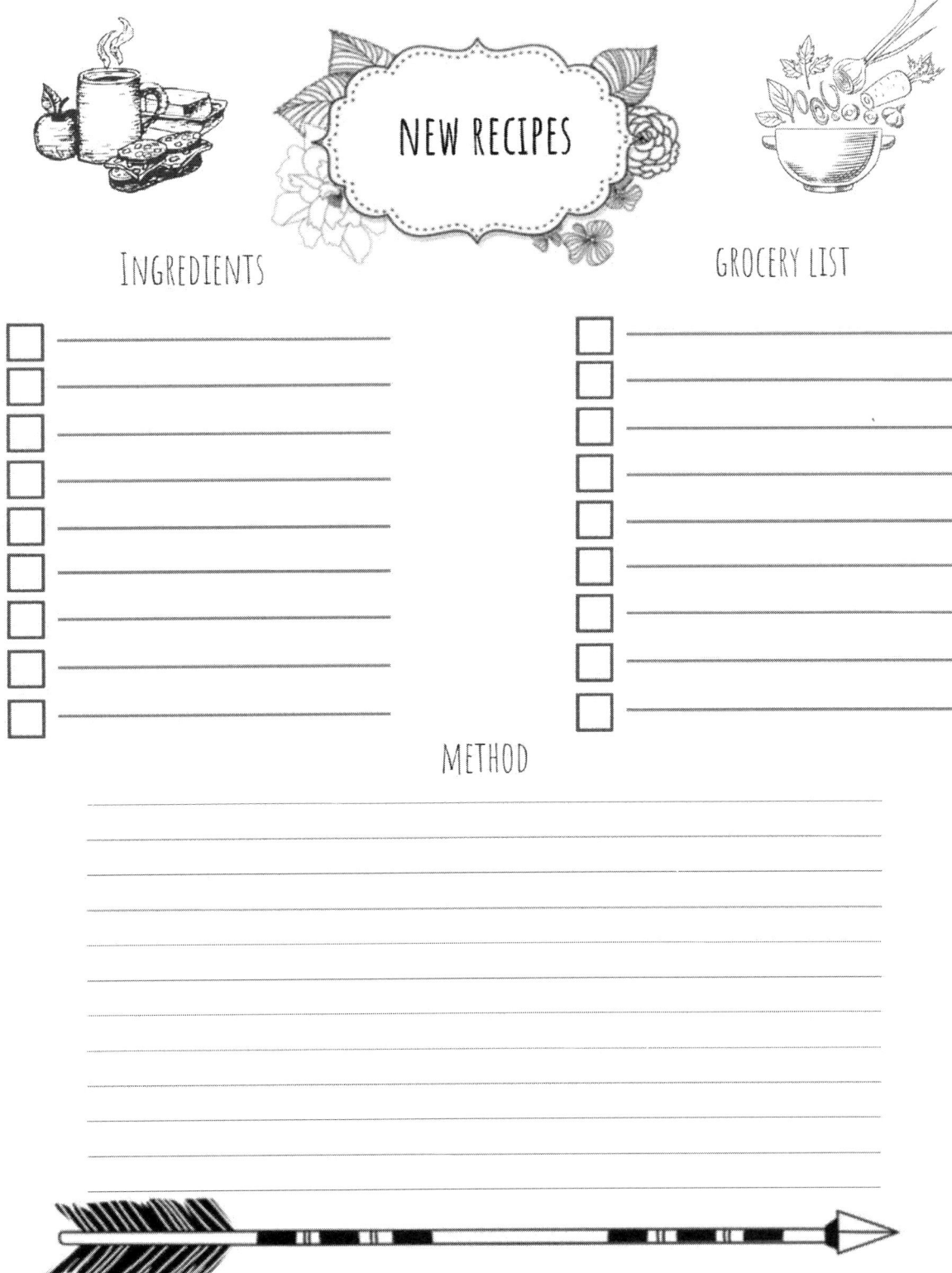

NEW RECIPES

Ingredients

- [ ]
- [ ]
- [ ]
- [ ]
- [ ]
- [ ]
- [ ]
- [ ]
- [ ]

Grocery List

- [ ]
- [ ]
- [ ]
- [ ]
- [ ]
- [ ]
- [ ]
- [ ]
- [ ]

Method

NEW RECIPES

Ingredients

- [ ] _____
- [ ] _____
- [ ] _____
- [ ] _____
- [ ] _____
- [ ] _____
- [ ] _____
- [ ] _____
- [ ] _____

Grocery List

- [ ] _____
- [ ] _____
- [ ] _____
- [ ] _____
- [ ] _____
- [ ] _____
- [ ] _____
- [ ] _____
- [ ] _____

Method

_____
_____
_____
_____
_____
_____
_____
_____

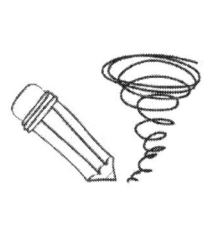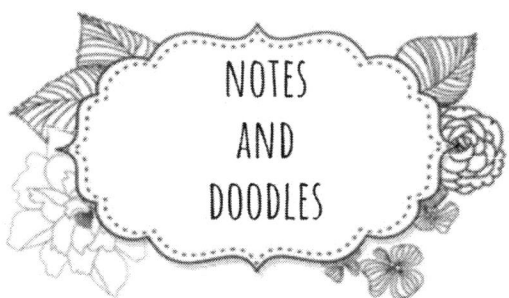

NOTES AND DOODLES

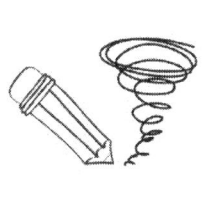
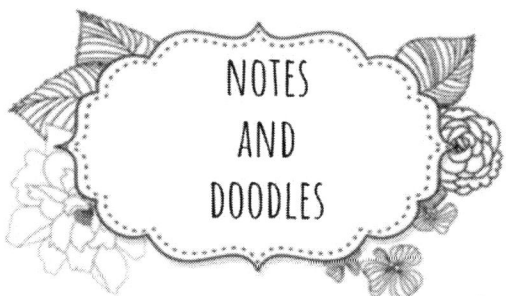

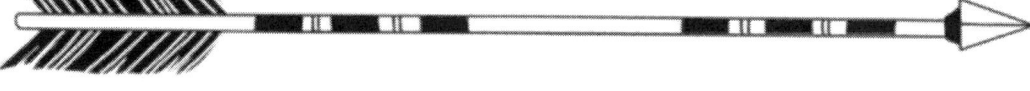

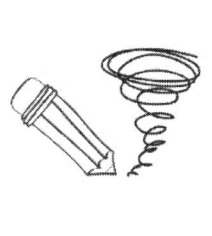 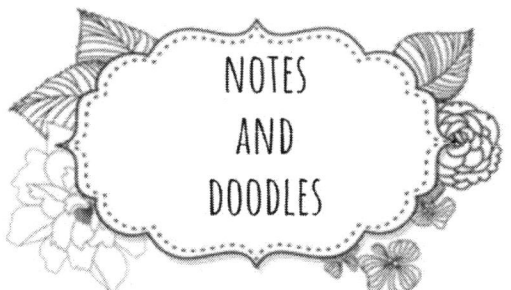 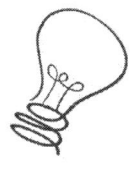

NOTES AND DOODLES

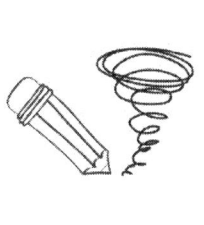 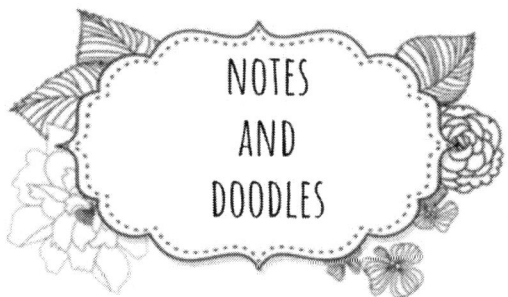 

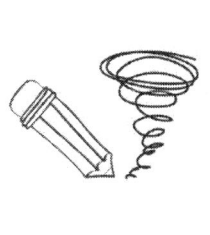
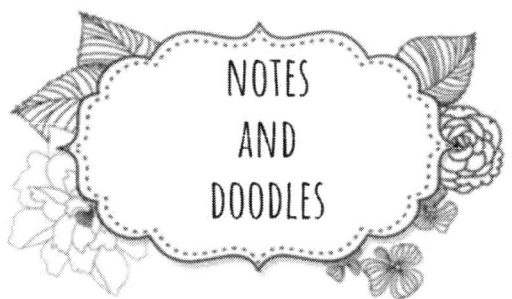

NOTES AND DOODLES

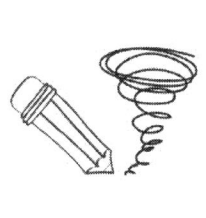
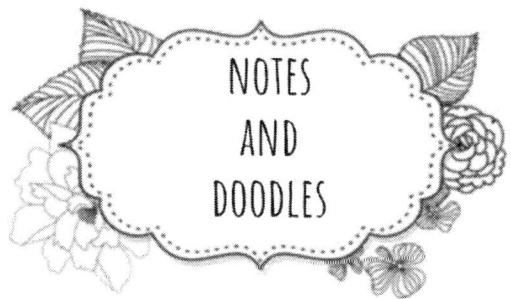

NOTES AND DOODLES

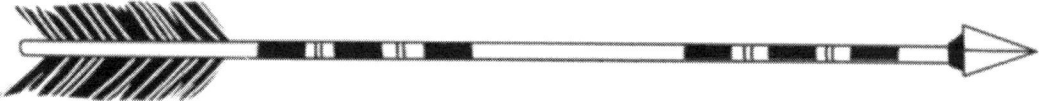

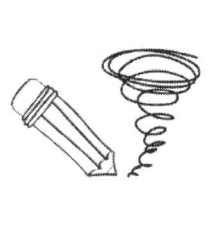 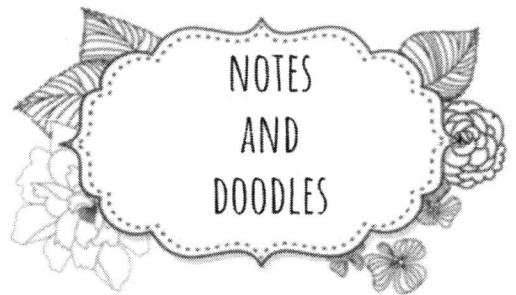 

NOTES AND DOODLES

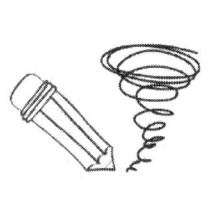 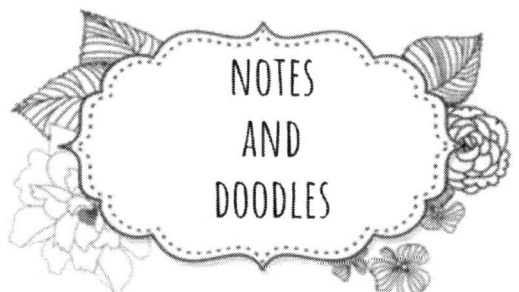 

NOTES AND DOODLES

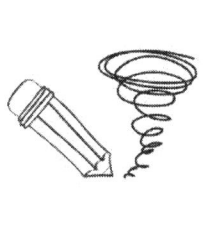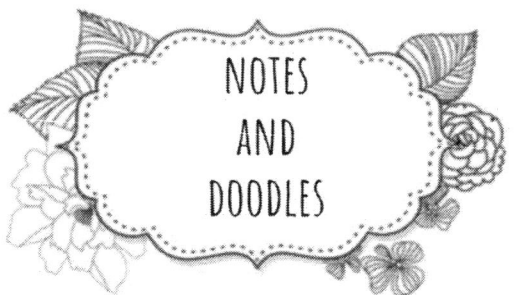

NOTES AND DOODLES

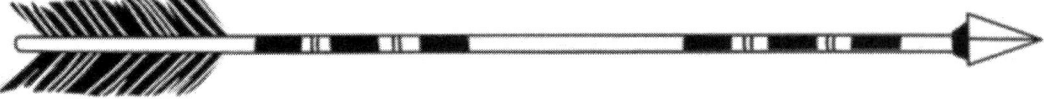

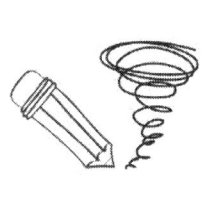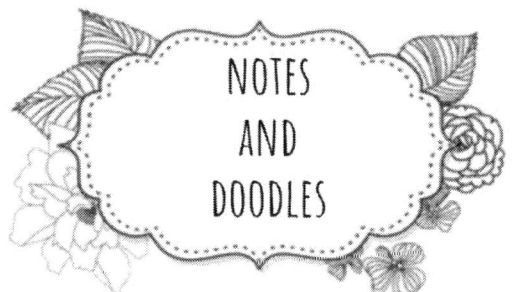

NOTES AND DOODLES

REMEMBER!

You'll be able to fill out your daily plan directly in the book or download a printable version at the link you see below to use the planner all year round as well.

https://BookHip.com/LGQXHHH

Journal created with the collaboration of **www.101planners.com**

Made in the USA
Monee, IL
26 December 2022

23668833R00085